The EEG of Mental Activities

Editors: D. Giannitrapani, Perry Point, Md.
L. Murri, Pisa

42 figures and 23 tables, 1988

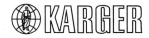

Basel · München · Paris ·
London · New York · New Delhi ·
Singapore · Tokyo · Sydney

Duilio Giannitrapani

PhD, Psychology Service, Veterans Administration Medical Center,
Perry Point, Md., USA

Luigi Murri

MD, Clinical Neurophysiology Service, Department of Neurology,
University of Pisa, Pisa, Italy

Library of Congress Cataloging-in-Publication Data
    The EEG of mental activities.
    Includes bibliographies and index.
    1. Electroencephalography.   2. Psychodiagnostics.
    3. Evoked potentials (Electrophysiology).   4. Higher nervous activity.
    I. Giannitrapani, Duilio.   II. Murri, Luigi, 1942–.
    [DNLM: 1. Electroencephalography.   2. Mental Disorders – diagnosis.   WL 150 E26]
    RC471.E33 1988   616.89′07′547   88-13168
    ISBN 3–8055–4812–5

Drug Dosage
    The authors and the publisher have exerted every effort to ensure that drug selection and
    dosage set forth in this text are in accord with current recommendations and practice at the
    time of publication. However, in view of ongoing research, changes in government regulations,
    and the constant flow of information relating to drug therapy and drug reactions, the reader is
    urged to check the package insert for each drug for any change in indications and dosage and
    for added warnings and precautions. This is particularly important when the recommended
    agent is a new and/or infrequently employed drug.

In memory of our dear friend and
distinguished scientist,

Leonide Goldstein

Contents

Individual Frequencies: Psychopathology

Preface

The kernel of this volume originates from a symposium, The EEG of Mental Activities, held in conjunction with the Annual Meeting of the Italian EEG Society in Viareggio in June 1986. During the process of gathering the manuscripts there have been many updates, revisions and changes in content that bring this volume to the present state of the art.

Contributions have been restricted to those utilizing EEG spectral analysis or evoked potential methodologies which have proven to be productive in the noninvasive study of physiological concomitants of higher cortical functions. It is already impossible to compose an all inclusive volume on this topic.

The reader, however, should not be misled into believing that the field has developed to the point in which all areas of mentation have been investigated. This is reflected in the titles of the sections which do not represent mutually exclusive categories but merely attempt to organize the available material into meaningful groups. The contributions selected offer a survey of some of the most recent methodological and theoretical approaches in this rapidly expanding field of neuroscience.

Duilio Giannitrapani
Luigi Murri

The Dementias

Giannitrapani, Murri (eds.), The EEG of Mental Activities,
pp. 1–25 (Karger, Basel 1988)

Event-Related Potentials' Changes in the Normal Presenium and in Patients with Initial Presenile Idiopathic Cognitive Decline[1]

Roberto Zappoli[2]

Second Neurological Institute, University of Florence, Florence, Italy

In recent years numerous studies have been published on the use of early, largely exogenous, stimulus-related potentials (EP) and late, largely endogenous, event-related potentials (ERP). They all consist of computer-averaged components of evoked potentials. These potentials, elicited with auditory, visual and somatosensory, nontarget or target and single or paired stimuli, have been used in evaluating normal decline with age and abnormal mental deterioration in elderly subjects.

A principal reason for interest in evoked potential research in this field is that it might contribute to the understanding of disorders of the central nervous system, particularly those at the subclinical level, as well as to the understanding of brain electrical activities associated with neurocognitive processes or the so-called higher mental functions. Over the past 2 decades numerous cognitively related ERP components reflecting different neuro- and psychophysiological activities (N1, P2, N1/P2 complex, N2, P3 or P3b, N4, SP, SW, BSP, CNV, etc.) have been discovered. The study of these ERP has expanded to such an extent that it can no longer be considered a unitary field of research.

Studies of the effects of aging and dementia on ERP were largely limited to the P300 (P3) and the contingent negative variation (CNV). The clinical utility of these kinds of ERP in the diagnosis of dementia and of

[1] A part of this work has been supported by Ministry of Education Research Fund for 1985.

[2] I am indebted to Miss Angela Versari for her skilfull technical assistance.

less profound cognitive deficits stressed by many authors [1–13] gives promise to an expanding role for clinical ERP applications. However, in order to use ERP components as a clinical tool, the changes due to normal aging, against which pathological deviations can be evaluated, must be well established. In general, collection of age-related normative data and studies of changes induced by processes of dementia and other neurocognitive disorders were limited until now to a small number of healthy subjects of different ages and to patients affected by a variety of forms of mental deterioration. Several discrepancies among the reported findings and data interpretation probably indicate that the effects of age and dementia on some ERP components are not ubiquitous and may vary with the experimental task.

The purpose of this article is to provide both an abbreviated review of selected papers dealing with the effects of age and primary processes of dementia on the most known types of ERP and personal observations especially focused on the presenium.

Slow Sensory and Long Latency ERP Components

Slow sensory and late ERP components [14] are dependent on the information content of stimuli. They appear only when a subject attends in some way to the stimuli and then only when a stimulus has meaning for the subject. The earliest slow ERP components usually appear within 150 ms after the stimulus, probably representing at the cortical level different aspects and stages of attentional-perceptual and discriminative functions and initial cognitive processing of stimuli which, when information processing is completed, lead to a decision.

There have been several studies of the changes induced by aging on the ERP components in the 80–150 ms latency range (especially the auditory N100 or N1 complex). These components, still sensitive to the physical properties of stimuli, were probably generated in the primary receiving area and with their apparently larger amplitude at the vertex essentially due to summation of the 2 temporal fields.

The so-called N1 component or 'vertex potential' of the auditory ERP is a complex composed of several relatively independent negative peaks [15]. It is generally accepted as a unitary component having a latency around 100 ms after stimulation. The auditory N1 varies in latency/amplitude with attended and non-attended stimuli and is thought to be a sign of early selective attention and habituation, sometimes referred to as 'channel selection' [16–18]. Gooding et al. [19] demonstrated that the N1 component, which is affected by tone intensity, was only different in latency by about 6 ms between normal young and old subjects with latency increase at the rate of 0.1 ms/year across the adult life span. Similar evidence of little but often nonsignificant slowing has been reported also by other researchers of N1 or 'vertex potential' for auditory stimuli [7, 20] and for visual and somatosensory ERP [1, 21–23]. The reported small age-related latency prolongation of auditory N1 was not observed by Pfefferbaum et al. [24–26]. Some significant decrease with age in amplitude of N1 was noted by Brent et al. [27] while Gooding et al. [19] found a reduction in the amplitude of the N1-P2 complex. For these 2 components differential effects of stimulus repetition were noted with age. The effect of repetition was essentially to reduce age-related amplitude differences between young and old in the later trial blocks [28].

The P200 (P2) peak which immediately follows auditory N1 also is considered to be in general an essentially exogenous component related to processes of selective attention and habituation. However, its topography is less dependent on stimulus modality, and its amplitude is not the largest over the sensory cortex. Latency of the auditory P2 component increased significantly with age at the rate of 0.7 ms/year [7, 19]. Old subjects demonstrated significantly smaller amplitude with differences in scalp distribution of P2 amplitude [7, 20, 27, 28]. Pfefferbaum et al. [24] noted that P2 in aged subjects was later but larger, and Dustman et al. [2] found no age-related changes for either N1 or P2 (N3, P3 in his nomenclature).

Some conflicting results were obtained by exploring in a small number of healthy young and old subjects the early components of the post-S1/S2 ERP evoked with paired auditory or visual stimuli of simple and choice warned reaction-time (RT) pardigms. In a selective attention task (Sternberg's memory search task, 82), Ford and her associates [29, 30, 43] demonstrated no significant age differences in the latency and amplitude of N1 and P2 ERP components for the warning auditory signals. This indicated that both young and old were attending selectively to the relevant channel at an equal level. With Sternberg's same short-term warned memory paradigm, Walrath and Hallman [31] observed no significant latency differences attributable to age in the post-S1 visual N150 and P240 ERP components. The ERP amplitude, however, was consistently smaller for the older subjects. No significant differences between ages were noted for the linear amplitude reduction in these components across trial blocks (habituation-like effects), but the older did show only slightly more consistent habituation than younger subjects.

The latency, amplitude and topographic distribution of the so-called cognitive late ERP components elicited with auditory stimuli, especially N2, P3, N4 and SW (slow negative after-wave), have all been shown to change as a function of age. The general trend in many situations, both simple and complex, consisted of increased latency and decreased amplitude with increasing age [20, 28, 32–35]. The same effect with age was observed for visual and somatosensory stimuli [2, 36, 37].

Prominent among cognitive ERP components is a late negative-positive complex comprising a brief and small negative wave (N200 or N2) followed immediately by a large positive composite wave (P300 or P3). All the waves of this complex are closely associated with one another, spatially and temporarily overlapped. They are, therefore, sometimes referred to as the N2-P3 complex even though they are related to different neurocognitive functions. When auditory stimuli are used in simple discrimination tasks, N2 is often small and not always easily identifiable because it is partly obscured by the surrounding positive components. N2 amplitude is consistent and readily detected when infrequent stimuli which deviate from the majority are administered. The amplitude of this 'mismatch negativity' (MMN) is inversely related to the frequency of the deviant stimuli, task relevant or not [38, 39]. Gooding et al. [19] noted a significant age-related increase in N2 latency (0.8 ms/year), while the N2-P3 amplitude decreased with age at the rate of 0.2 μV/year. Brent et al. [27], using auditory stimuli, also reported a longer latency with age for the N2 component of the 'vertex' potential but no age-related changes in the amplitude of this badly identifiable component.

P300 or P3 is a positive 'endogenous' wave peaking about 300 ms after infrequent task-relevant stimuli. Its scalp topography and behavior do not depend on physical stimulus properties per se but on their 'meaning' in the context of the task. It has been suggested that P3 is related to 'perception and cognition' and seems to express the conclusion of the stimulus processing sequence. Adopting different kinds of stimulation in more or less complex discrimination and multiple decision tasks or go/no-go situations [for reviews see ref. 40, 41], at least 2 separate and relatively independent components with different properties and scalp distribution have been identified: P3a or P270 and P3b the 'true P3' [37, 42].

Whatever the true significance of P3 and its components, several studies [7, 8, 12, 19, 20, 28, 32, 34, 35] have shown that auditory P3 latency increases with aging by about 1.0–1.8 ms/year. Most reports indicated that the relationship between auditory P3 latency and age is linear although Brown et al. [44] argued that this correlation is nonsignificant below 45 years of age. They suggested that the best fit between P3 latency and age is curvilinear. P3 was shown to have also an effect age-related to a visual task. In that case the best relationship was not linear but curvilinear [45]. The relationship between P300 latency and age was found to be steeper for visual than auditory targets with the relationship for the somatosensory stimulus being steeper yet [34, 35, 37]. Even the latency of P270 (P3a) increased significantly with age [37].

Different results were obtained regarding the relationship between age and P3 amplitude. Gooding et al. [19] reported a decrease with age in the N2-P3 peak-to-peak amplitude, and Smith et al. [28] noted that in younger subjects the P3 wave for the infrequent tone was almost twice as large as in older subjects. Pfefferbaum et al. [25, 26] showed that old subjects had smaller P3s at P_z and larger ones at F_z when compared to the young. Brent et al. [27] reported smaller P3 in older than in younger subjects at both central and parietal recording sites.

In general, anterior-posterior amplitude differences of several components, especially auditory N1-P2, N2 and P3, have consistently distinguished young from old persons. In contrast to younger subjects, who exhibit larger ERP in central and parietal regions for auditory and somatosensory stimuli and a marked negative-to-positive gradient from frontal to parietal electrodes, older subjects have a more equipotential distribution of amplitude across the whole scalp with reduction in frontal activity [20, 28]. Other investigators found no significant age differences in P3 amplitude [37].

Some contrasting data were collected for a few normal elderly subjects regarding the effect of age on the post-S1/S2 P3 components elicited with paired stimuli in simple and choice constant foreperiod RT experiments. Marsh [46], utilizing signaled tasks and speed instructions, reported a lack of age differences in P3 latency and a significant reduction of P3 amplitude with increasing age. During performance on Sternberg's tasks, Ford et al. [29, 30, 81] noted an increased latency with age of the P3 to the warning auditory signal while the amplitude and scalp distribution of P3 were not different for young and elderly subjects.

Podlesny and Dustman [47], using signaled simple and choice RT tasks, recorded an age reduction in P3 amplitude, but no effects of age were observed on P3 latency. Amplitude reduction, especially in centroparietal areas, and higher mean latency of P3 to visual S1 were measured by Tecce et al. [48–50] both in older and the oldest in comparison with younger groups of subjects tested with a simple constant foreperiod RT task. The relationship between P3 and RT was always a complex one and deserves further consideration [46, 51].

There are many discrepancies among the reported findings and data interpretation of the age-related changes of P3 latency, amplitude and scalp topography, probably due to the variety of experimental designs, recording procedures and methods of measurement adopted generally for small groups of healthy elderly subjects. The latency of the P3 component elicited with simple discrimination and go/no-go tasks seems to be the most effective electrophysiological measure for objectively evaluating variations in mental status associated with age, various forms of dementia and other neurocognitive disorders [3, 4, 6–8, 12].

According to Squires et al. [7] e.g. the average P3 latency of the demented patients exceeded the mean value of age-matched normal subjects by 3.61 SD. Using the criterion of P3 latency in excess of 2 SD, 80% of the demented patients were successfully identified. P3 latency thus seems to provide a very sensitive measure for differentiating primary and secondary organic dementia from functional disorders such as depression or other disorders of movement or linguistic skills.

More recently, a negative wave peaking at about 400 ms (N4) was reported to be related to 'semantic incongruity' of sentences [52, 53]. A semantically appropriate word presented in a larger typeface elicited a P3 without N4. This suggests that deviation from semantic context was required for elicitation of N4. With semantic tasks the N4 wave appeared with greater latency in the elderly [54].

Some tasks with rare, novel or complex unpaired stimuli frequently elicit a long-duration slow wave (SW) which begins as early as 180 ms, peaks between 500 and 700 ms and may persist for 1 s or more following the evoking stimulus [34, 55, 56]. As in the case of the late positive complex, the SW appears to comprise several waves and especially an early (500–650 ms) and a later (500–700 ms) component. The early wave reflects a negative-to-positive gradient from frontal to more posterior electrodes (frontal negative after-wave). The later component shows a negative focus at the vertex, but in general the midline distribution of the SW is typically negative at F_z, positive at P_z and about 0 at C_z [57, 58]. In particular, the early frontal negative component of the SW, like the early component of the CNV or the so-called O-wave, is thought to be associated with 'orienting' [55–58], i.e. with processes subsequent to stimulus evaluation in the context of the current trial.

As in the case of the fronto-central negativity of the late sustained potential (SP) of Pfefferbaum et al. [24–26], the SW frontal negativity was either markedly reduced or absent in elderly subjects [20, 28]. In addition, this reduction or absence of the frontal negative after-wave with aging means an absence of the negative-to-positive gradient that characterized the younger subjects [20, 24, 26, 28]. According to Smith et al. [20, 28], these age differences in the SW components can be interpreted as reflecting a process of selective cortical aging involving essentially the frontal areas of the brain which are associated with the more typical perceptual and performance deficits of the elderly.

Current Research

Using a standard S1-2 sec-S2 CNV-RT (motor-response) paradigm, during the past year or so we have carried out studies [13, 59, 82] of several post-S1 (a click) ERP components (N1, P2 and P3) in a group of 20 selected very healthy subjects: 10 young adults (age range 25–33 years; $\overline{X}$ 28.3) and 10 presenile subjects (age range 55–64 years; $\overline{X}$ 59.6). In addition, the same ERP components were measured in a group of 10 subjects (age range 50–65 years; $\overline{X}$ 58.6) with initial presenile idiopathic cognitive decline (PICD) and presumptive diagnosis of an early stage of presenile dementia. They, however, did not meet DSM-III criteria for dementia. The 10 patients with PICD and without neurological or auditory problems (Hachinski's ischemic index equal to or lower than 5) complained mainly of moderate loss of memory function and complex cognitive processes, of reduced attention, concentration and performance especially in the divided attention situations, and of sporadic brief episodes of amnesia or simple anomia. EEG, post-S1 ERP and CNV components were recorded from F_z, C_3, C_z, C_4, P_3, P_z and P_4 referred to linked mastoid electrodes.

Electro-oculogram, S1, S2 and RT were also recorded. Details of the methods and statistical analysis have been reported in previous papers [13, 59, 82]. The main results were the following:

N1. At all recording sites, in comparison with younger normal subjects there was either a significant increased mean latency of N1 to S1 in PICD patients or a significant mean amplitude reduction of this component in both the PICD and normal presenile groups. No significant group differences were found in the scalp distribution of mean latency of N1, while in all 3 groups there was a pattern of higher mean latency of N1 to the warning signal in parietal areas compared to the other fronto-central locations ($p < 0.05$). We are not aware that these between-group significant N1 amplitude differences at all leads, especially at C_z, have been described by other researchers.

P2. In comparison with the younger subjects, significant increased latency of the P2 to S1 component was observed in different leads in normal presenile and PICD groups.

P3. Regarding the post-S1 P3 component, the mean latency and amplitude in the presenile subjects were significantly higher at parietal recording sites as compared to the other fronto-central leads. No significant differences were measured in the scalp distribution of P3 mean latency and amplitude in either young or PICD groups. Significant between-group differences were recorded at all leads but especially in parietal areas for P3 latencies which, in comparison with the young subjects, were longer in the presenile group ($p < 0.05$ or < 0.02) and increased further in PICD patients ($p < 0.01$). In the parietal leads also the P3 amplitude was significantly augmented in PICD patients as compared to younger normal subjects. Regarding effects of repetition on all the post-S1 ERP taken into account, latencies, amplitudes and scalp topography in the 2 groups of normal subjects did not differ significantly across the consecutive 4 blocks of 8 averaged trials (32 artifact-free responses for each subject). In the group of PICD patients instead, progressive increased latencies and reduced amplitudes across the last 2 blocks of responses (habituation-like effect) were noted.

RT. (Operant motor response: S2 interruption). In contrast to the findings obtained for young subjects, prolonged mean RT were observed in the normal presenile group and especially in PICD patients. The difference in mean RT between the young and presenile groups failed to reach statistical significance ($p = 0.089$), while it was statistically significant ($p < 0.05$) between young subjects and PICD patients.

Steady Potential Shifts

Most studies of steady potential shifts (SPS; 14) in aging subjects with normal mental status and behavior or in patients with different forms of neurocognitive disorders have been focused on the so-called Bereitschafts-potential (BSP or readiness potential) and the CNV. These terms denote a class of complex negative slow potential shifts lasting for a second or more. Several researchers in this field have reported results often with discrepancies which very probably were due to the variety of experimental designs, recording procedures and methods of analysis adopted.

The BSP consists of a slowly increasing negative shift 1–2 s prior to movement, rapidly followed by a positive deflection after the start of the movement [60]. It comprises at least 3 components [61]. Deecke et al. [62] noted a gradual decrease of BSP with increasing age past 40 and almost no potential in subjects over 60 years. These findings could account for lower amplitudes in elderly subjects of the late CNV component, the so-called 'E' or 'P' (expectancy or preparatory) component, elicited by Loveless and Sandford [63] and employing long interstimulus intervals (ISI) up to 15 s. In contrast to the BSP which sometimes occurred as a positive shift in centro-parietal areas for subjects over 60 years, the true motor potential was essentially constant across ages [20, 62]. With a procedure used in the voluntary movement conditions that does not closely replicate the method of Deecke et al. [60, 62], Loveless [64] felt unable to demonstrate significant aging effects on BSP amplitude.

Another example of a SPS in the CNV first described by Walter et al. [65]. This long-lasting surface negative shift, a true mosaic of overlapping components related to different neuro- and psychophysiological functions by now sufficiently known, developed between the time of a warning signal (S1) and a second 'imperative' stimulus (S2) which demanded some form of response: operant motor response, inhibition of a motor response, or a decision [56, 65, 66].

The CNV was thought to reflect essentially arousal, attention, concentration, short-term memory and motivation necessary in preparation to act. CNV is affected by many cognitive factors including distraction, anticipation of information, ambiguity and task difficulty, personality, etc., and by noncognitive factors such as stimulus intensity, modality and timing, RT and magnitude of movement, fatigue, age, various types of drugs and neuro-psychic disorders, etc. [for review see ref. 56, 66]. If the S1-S2 interval is extended beyond 2 s or more, mainly 2 overlapping negative waves with different topographies and responses to experimental factors compose the CNV.

The earlier of these, often called the 'orienting' or 'O-waves', is a frontally maximum negative wave following S1, depends on the properties of the warning signal and is very likely an instance of the frontal negative after-wave (SW, see above) to S1. The second late CNV component, which has been called the 'expectancy' or 'preparatory (E or P) wave', is a centrally maximum negative shift preceding S2 and reaching maximal negativity just prior to the end of ISI. This late CNV component reflects the process of preparation to act and, in the case of an operant motor response to S2, is probably an instance of the BSP (see above).

According to these interpretative hypotheses of the 2 principal CNV components, in some instances it was observed that with a short ISI the CNV is merely a composite of 2 separate negative overlapped waves. Rohrbaugh et al. [56] synthesized a CNV-like waveform from ERPs accompanying unassociated events: the essentially frontal slow negative after-wave (SW) following unpaired auditory or visual stimuli, the BSP preceding self-initiated finger movements and the ERP to another unpaired stimulus. A number of studies have investigated age-related CNV changes, and several authors have reported that in older individuals the development of this complex cortical bioelectric event is altered in both magnitude and shape [10, 48–50, 63, 66–68].

A brief overview of the very few studies on CNV parameters and RT changes induced by aging shows that no evidence has yet been found for demonstrating a precise constant relationship between the brain involutional processes and the CNV complex with its various components and related cognitive activities. For example, in studies that have utilized fixed short S1-S2 intervals, where CNV appears as a unitary wave, no clear age differences have been noted [63, 69, 70]. For longer ISI, however, the preparatory pre-S2 component (P-wave), similar to the BSP recorded in older subjects by Deecke et al. [62], is reported to be either diminished [71] or even absent in the elderly [63]. Moreover, the latter authors reported that about 1 s after the warning signal early CNV components ('orienting' or O-wave) appeared which were larger in the younger group of normal subjects.

No differences were observed by Schaie and Syndulko [71] in the amplitudes of the CNV O-wave, but they did find a delayed latency for the elderly. Michalewski et al. [72], in control situations using a standard CNV paradigm or in distraction conditions, noted on all occasions in the elderly a significant amplitude reduction of the P-wave only in frontal areas, while vertex and parietal amplitudes were comparable between younger and elderly subjects. Nakamura et al. [67], adopting a standard CNV paradigm, noted that when a motor response to S2 was required CNV decreased and RT increased with age, and these age-related CNV/RT changes probably depend on an impaired mechanism for sustaining attention and dysfunction in memory processes.

A line of research followed by Tecce et al. [48–50] has been based on the relationship between CNV amplitude and distraction and divided attention situations (short-term memory tasks) during ISI that interfere with the selection of the relevant information processing and result in a marked decrement of CNV amplitude and prolonged RT. This CNV distraction effect is followed in the subsequent unexpected control trials by a supranormal increase of the CNV activity (CNV rebound effect: CNVR) which is significantly and selectively diminished in frontocentral areas of elderly subjects. This phenomenon was interpreted as reflecting a weakened ability among older individuals to switch attention sets mediated in part by frontal brain areas. In this respect, the elderly resemble Alzheimer patients who have no CNVR [11]. CNVR effect was absent in the 14 Alzheimer patients, mostly elderly, examined by Tecce et al. [11]. According to these researchers the finding of a poorly developed CNVR in a normal elderly person may be a precursor sign of senile dementia.

Under baseline conditions and when distracting stimuli were introduced also, Rizzo et al. [9] found in 8 patients with presenile dementia significantly reduced CNV activity and longer RT. Using a task similar to that employed by Tecce et al. [48–50, 68], Michalewski et al. [72] independently produced similar results and, in addition, they noted that even with a standard S1-S2 CNV paradigm the frontal CNV for the older persons were reduced compared in the young group. These authors pointed out that this overall reduction in frontal CNV activity in the aged suggests a process of selective aging in the frontal lobe probably related to a loss in cellular and dendritic mass of the frontal premotor and association cortical areas.

In some studies, age differences in CNV were limited to a difficult task [69]. In other studies, no substantial age-CNV association was found [30, 73]. Surprisingly, Podlesny and Dustman [47], with simple and choice warned RT tasks and speed instructions, claim to have observed in elderly subjects a paradoxical increase in CNV activity and slower RT, possibly indicating weaker inhibitory function. As noted earlier, several apparent conflicts between the reported findings probably indicate that the effects of age and cognitive decline on the CNV complex are not ubiquitous and may vary with the experimental task. Moreover, on the basis of these observations, it appears clearly that the effects of age and dementing diseases on CNV activity, until now, have been examined in a too limited number of normal subjects and patients with impaired mental function of various degree and age of onset, for the most part the very elderly, sometimes with discrepancies among the reported findings and data interpretation probably depending, for one reason, on the numerous kinds of tasks adopted.

Additional CNV Findings

Very recently we carried out a new method of analysis of the CNV complex, designed to investigate eventual differences in several CNV components and RT between either healthy young adults and presenile subjects, or patients with PICD and initial mild-moderate-severe presenile Alzheimer-type dementia (PAD). All of the 7 patients with PAD (age range 55–65 years; $\overline{X}$ 60.8) examined till the present time presented a progressive cognitive impairment that met the DSM-III criteria for presenile primary dementia.

The purpose was to collect additional normative data in healthy subjects and patients with initial forms of presenile cognitive deficits in the hope of providing practical and objective measures of those psychophysiological conditions expressed by the CNV activity in the normal presenium and possibly useful clinically for identifying the early stages of presenile neurological diseases affecting cognitive processes. To this end the already mentioned simple S1-2 sec-S2-RT paradigm was used, and each artifact-free response recorded with 7 leads was analyzed separately at 4 independent temporal window-areas (WA) of 200 ms duration corresponding to the most important and known CNV components.

During the ISI and the post-S2 CNV resolution, the positions of the WAs were: WA1 500–700 ms post-S1, the 'O-wave'; WA2 1100–1300 ms, the N1200, the so-called 'saddle'; WA3 1,800–2,000 ms pre-S2, the 'P-wave'; WA4 400–600 ms after S2 interruption, variable relative to RT duration, the CNV resolution (fig. 1). The method of the WA of 200 ms duration ($\mu V \cdot s$), unlike other methods of CNV activity analysis, reduces considerably the between-subjects variability. For measurements we adopted either a classic method of averaging (fig. 1, 2) or a method of spatio-temporal topographic CNV activity mapping (more details on the methods and data analysis have been reported in previous papers) [13, 59, 82]. For illustrative purposes CNV/RT grand averages were constructed across each group of subjects (shown in fig. 1, 2). The main results were as follows:

In the normal subjects, significant young-presenile differences were found in the early and late (O-wave and P-wave) CNV components. These were smaller in the older subjects, essentially in centro-parietal areas (fig. 1a, b). A progressive amplitude reduction only in frontal leads between O-wave (WA1) and P-wave (WA3) was characteristic in the presenile group (fig. 1b, 2a). These subjects showed also relatively flat CNV waveshapes of low amplitude in all centro-parietal areas (fig. 2a). This waveform was similar to that described by Loveless and Sandford [63] in more aged healthy subjects. The presenile group, as a whole, performed a little worse than young subjects, even if no significance between group differences was observed in the mean RT values. These findings suggest that the statistically significant changes of CNV activity, recorded in our presenile subjects without appreciable deficits of behavioral and mental performances, could be signs of early stages of brain involutional processes related to minimal and subclinical decrement of orienting, attentiveness and response preparation capabilities.

Compared with the presenile subjects who showed a progressive decline in amplitude between WA1 and WA3 only in frontal leads, in PICD patients a significant decrement of the late 'P' CNV component measured with WA3 was observed in all recording sites, especially in central regions (fig. 1c, 2b). PICD patients showed prolonged RT, but the differences compared to the presenile group reached no statistical significance. They

---

Fig. 1. Criteria used for CNV/RT measurements. Each measure (e.g. the WAs in F_z and C_z marked in black) is a mean voltage over 200 ms ($\mu V \cdot s$) respectively at 500–700, 1,100–1,300, 1,800–2,000 ms post-S1, and 400–600 ms after S2 interruption (variable relative to RT duration). *a* Grand average across 10 normal young adults ($\overline{X} = 28.3$ years); 320 trials (4 blocks of 8 consecutive averaged trials from each subject); mean RT 210 ms. *b* Grand average of 10 normal presenile subjects ($\overline{X} = 59.6$ years); 320 trials and mean RT 275 ms. *c* Grand average of 10 patients with PICD ($\overline{X} = 58.6$ years); 320 trials and mean RT 335 ms. *a–c* Mean latency of N1 and P3 to S1 at P_z respectively 110, 330 ms; 115, 340 ms and 130, 335 ms. More details in Zappoli et al. [13, 59, 82].

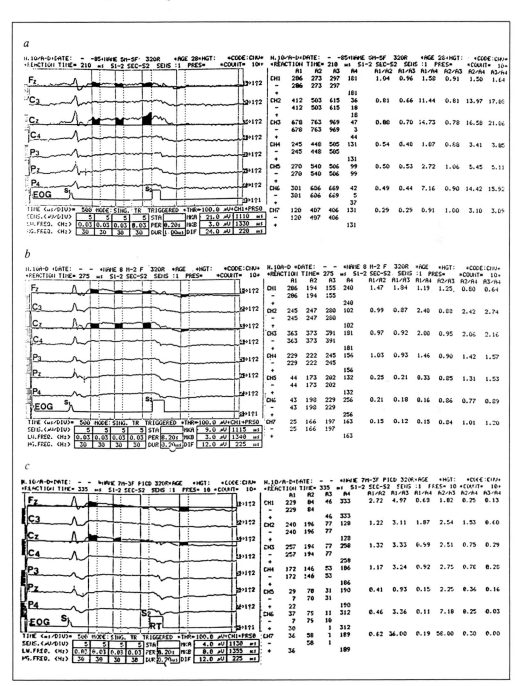

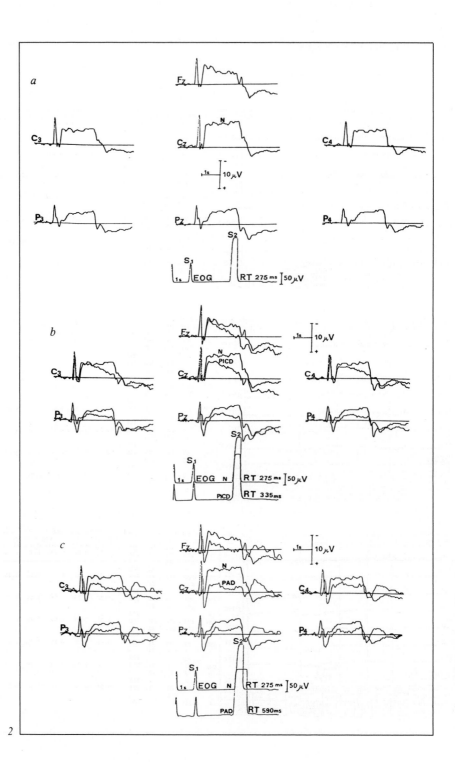

were statistically significant between the PICD and young group. The diffused marked reduction of the P-wave in these patients, which correlated significantly with longer RT [13], may be indicative of a difficulty in sustaining a sufficient level of attention and preparation to respond properly to imperative signals [63, 74].

With the exception of a small post-S1 orienting component in fronto-central areas, in PAD patients the CNV activity on the whole was practically absent (fig. 2c). PAD patients, moreover, had highly significant prolonged RT compared with the other 3 groups of subjects. The lack of a CNV activity in our demented patients probably depends on their inability to recognize the warning significance of the first signal (S1). They responded with enormous delay only to the second imperative signal which means they were not waiting for S2. Four of the 7 PAD patients showed in several blocks of 8 artifact-free averaged responses with typical large post-imperative negative variations (PINV). In the across-subject grand average this particular bioelectric event was quite evident (fig. 2c). PINV is frequently observable in the psychiatric population, but it is not specific to a single diagnosis even if it appears to be a sensitive index of psychopathological morbidity [75].

Discussion and Conclusions

All research, reviewed in this paper, on ERP changes due to aging processes and other forms of neurocognitive and performance capacity decline permits a brief discussion and a number of conclusions.

In spite of some contrasting data reported in the literature [30, 43, 81], in our research the post-S1 N1 and P2 components, evoked with a standard paired auditory stimuli RT task and speed instructions, showed several significant amplitude and latency changes in healthy presenile subjects and PICD patients in comparison with the young adults. Among the findings recorded were essentially a diffuse mean amplitude reduction of N1 to S1, both in presenile and PICD groups, and a significant slowing of N1 and, in fronto-central areas, of P2 components in PICD patients compared to the 2 groups of normal subjects.

We are not aware that these changes of the post-warning stimulus N1 and P2 ERP components have been described by other researchers. If these

---

Fig. 2. a Grand average waveform across 10 normal (N) presenile subjects (320 trials; mean RT 275 ms). *b* Superimposition of the grand average waveforms across 10 normals (N) and 10 patients with PICD (320 trials; mean RT 335 ms). *c* Superimposition of the grand average waveforms across 10 normals (N) and 7 patients with PAD (224 trials; mean RT 590 ms). In the PAD group a clear PINV appears after S2.

results are confirmed in a larger number of subjects and if we accept the interpretative hypotheses of these two ERP components put forward by Hillyard et al. [16, 17], our data would suggest that already in the normal presenium and still more in PICD patients there is probably a more or less marked deficit of early selective attention and habituation performances.

We also noted significance between group differences in mean latencies of P3 to S1 which was longer in all leads, especially in the parietal areas, in the presenile group and still longer in PICD patients. These results agree with the data obtained with S1-S2 task in healthy old or very old subjects by Ford et al. [29, 30, 43, 81] and Tecce et al. [49, 50]. According to these researchers the generalized increase in latency of P3 to S1 in their subjects appears to reflect impairment in attention functions and stimulus evaluation capacity. This hypothesis appears to be acceptable as the P3 prolongation was more marked in our PICD patients who complained mainly of reduced attention, concentration and loss of memory. Regarding the slowing of post-S1 P3, it must be emphasized that a significant increase in latency of this component, especially in parietal recording sites, was found to be present in our normal subjects in the presenium while other investigators generally describe it in subjects of much more advanced age.

These results, together with those obtained with different kinds of task-relevant unpaired stimuli eliciting the P3 ERP component, have confirmed what behavioral studies have been indicating for decades, i.e. that the central processing time is slower in the older brain. Squire et al. [7] concluded that cognitive deficit in the elderly expressed by the progressive age-dependent P3 prolongation, may be accounted for by slower decision time. They demonstrated that the P3 is one of the most effective electrophysiological measures for evaluating variation in mental status associated with dementing diseases. Dementia exacerbates the effects of normal aging so that demented patients have much greater latency P3 waves. Indeed, the P3 can be a useful measure to identify early stages and different forms of dementia. The real functional significance and the specific causes of the P3 prolongation related to aging processes, however, remain to be determined. This determination is crucial to understanding the meaning of the reports of P3 increased latency in dementing diseases [3, 6–8, 20].

CNV-RT performances provide useful information in the study of the effects of aging and dementing illness on neurocognitive processes. In general, CNV activity decreases and RT increases with age, and dementia sharply emphasizes this trend which is particularly evident when the attention or concentration are disturbed during ISI, e.g. when divided-procedures are utilized [9–11, 13, 48–50, 59, 66, 68, 72]. Concerning the more important and known CNV components, waveform analysis of CNV in our subjects [13, 59, 82] indicated that the main age effects were found in the early O-wave and late P-wave and that the group differences were further increased in PICD and especially in PAD patients (fig. 1, 2).

The O-wave, measured with the WA1 (fig. 1), was significantly larger at central and parietal leads in the young compared with the presenile subjects and the 2 groups of patients. It is generally recognized that the O-wave of the CNV, like the slow negative after-waves labeled SW [55, 58], reflects behaviorally oriented processes such as perception and attention. The decreased amplitude of these 2 bioelectrical events was interpreted in the elderly and in dementing diseases, as the effect of a reduced cortical excitability and/or of difficulty in sustaining adequate arousal/attention levels [10, 11, 13, 20, 24, 25, 28, 50, 72].

Regarding the late CNV P-wave, very likely reflecting preparatory strategy and especially motor preparation processes [63, 74, 76], larger amplitude was measured in all leads of our young group compared with presenile subjects. A progressive amplitude reduction of CNV complex only in frontal areas between the WA1 and WA3, the latter reaching the lowest point (fig. 1b, 2a), and a relatively flat CNV waveshape in the other recording sites were characteristic in the presenile subjects' group. A clear progressive amplitude decrement of CNV complex from WA1 to WA3, diffused at all recording sites but especially over the fronto-central areas, was observed in our patients with PICD (fig. 1c, 2b). In patients with PAD, the WA3 and the CNV activity on the whole were practically absent (fig. 2c). Relevant to this also was the significant negative correlation found in both groups of patients between the WA3 and RT: the smaller the WA3 the longer the RT [13].

These data are in accordance with the hypothesis of Loveless and Sandford [63] and Gaillard [74] that the smaller amplitude of the CNV P-wave in association with slow RT may be indicative of a difficulty in sustaining, over the entire task duration, a sufficient level of attention and preparation essential for responding properly to imperative signals. This condition could be one of the features of the performance deficits in the elderly and patients with dementia.

The lack of a persistent, consistent CNV activity in all leads and the very abnormal increase of the RT in PAD patients were probably due to the fact that our patients with presenile primary dementia, in spite of repeated instructions, did not recognize the warning significance of the first signal and responded with enormous delay only to the second imperative signal. They were not waiting for S2. These data, together with those of Tecce et al. [11] on the absence of the CNV rebound effect in older Alzheimer's patient, suggest that these CNV-RT changes probably depend on a severely impaired mechanism for sustaining attention and marked dysfunction in memory processes.

Our normal presenile subjects, in addition to the significant reduction of the P-wave only in F_z, showed relatively flat square-topped CNV wave-shapes of low amplitude in all centro-parietal areas. This waveform was similar to that described by Loveless and Sandford [63] in more aged healthy subjects. A nearly equipotential amplitude distribution across the whole scalp was found by Smith et al. [20, 28] in older persons also for the so-called SW (see above).

All of these findings, especially the amplitude reduction of the CNV P-wave only in the F_z recording site [72], the CNV rebound effect significantly and selectively diminished in fronto-central regions [48–50] and the decrement of other types of ERPs (P3, SP, SW) elicited in frontal areas by a variety of tasks [6, 20, 24–26, 28], induced Smith et al. [20, 28], Michalewski et al. [72] and Tecce et al. [48–50] to put forward a hypothesis. It was that the reduced frontal activity in healthy elderly persons may be caused by an enhanced selective aging process in the frontal premotor and association cortices linked to performance deficits observable in these subjects. According to Tecce et al. [10, 11], the finding of a poorly developed CNV rebound effect in the apparently normal elderly could be a precursor sign of senile dementia.

As a whole, all these data on the age-related changes of different ERP over the frontal regions are in agreement with the ideas of Albert and Kaplan [77]. Having reviewed the relevant literature in neuropsychology, they concluded that perceptual and performance deficits in the elderly are suggestive of involvement of the frontal cortex. Neuroanatomical changes, with more marked neuronal loss in prefrontal and parieto-temporal association cortical areas, have frequently been reported in the elderly brain [78–80]. According to Smith et al. [20, 28] behavioral, neuroanatomical and ERP data are converging to suggest a deficit with age especially in the frontal lobes.

If we accept this hypothesis, the reduced amplitude of the WA3 (P-wave) only in F_z and the relatively flat waveshape with smaller amplitude of the CNV in the centro-parietal areas, observed in our presenile subjects, would point out that such presumed selective cortical aging may start in the presenium without being revealed by particular behavioral and mental deficits. These CNV changes may be signs of early stages of brain involutional processes, especially of frontal associative and premotor cortices, related to an initial minimal and subclinical decrement of orienting, attentiveness and response preparation capabilities.

With reference to this, we think it is useful to mention that Ford and Pfefferbaum [81] were the first to observe, with CT scan examinations, a decrease in brain tissue linked with longer latency P3 waves. However, only one of our patients with PICD had a moderately diffuse cortical atrophy. All the other patients of this group had CT scans within the normal limits. All patients with PAD showed a more or less severely diffuse cortical-subcortical atrophy with CT scan and NMR examinations.

It is also of some importance to note that 4 of the 7 patients with PAD showed typical PINVs in several trial blocks. PINV has been frequently observed in psychiatric patients, but it is not specific to a single diagnosis even if it appears to be a sensitive index of psychopathology, particularly schizophrenia [75].

In conclusion, ERP and especially P3 and CNV-RT performances are without doubt sensitive to age-dependent cognitive slowing as well as to disease-induced cognitive impairment. From the few ERP studies mentioned, practically the 2 promising theoretical developments in the understanding of brain functioning, effects of aging and other forms of mental decline that have resulted are the distraction-arousal hypothesis and the controlled-automatic attention model [10]. In our experience the effects on post-S1 ERP, CNV activity and RT of aging and of the impairment of neurocognitive processes essentially related to attention, concentration and memory functions induced the more or less marked and characteristic changes observed in the majority of the limited number of normal subjects and patients so far examined.

In addition, our results show that already in the normal presenium there may exist substantial differences of several CNV components associated with a moderate increase in RT. The changes of CNV-RT performances in PICD and PAD patients also appeared to be fairly characteristic. If these changes are confirmed in a larger sample of healthy subjects and PICD and PAD patients and show sufficient stability, they could have considerable practical importance for clinical and research applications. One end could be the use of these noninvasive methods of observing neurophysiological events in the CNS for identifying the initial stages of brain involutional processes and the precursor signs of presenile neurological diseases affecting cognitive functions. A prolonged follow-up study in more cases, supplied with neuroradiological, neurochemical, neuropsychological, laboratory and clinical examinations, will be able or not to confirm our promising preliminary results.

References

1   Straumanis, J.S.; Schagass, C.; Schwartz, M.: Visually evoked cerebral response changes associated with chronic brain syndromes and aging. J. Geront. *20:* 498–506 (1965).

2   Dustman, R.E.; Schentenberg, T.; Beck, E.C.: The development of the evoked response as a diagnostic and evaluative procedure; in Karrer, Developmental psychophysiology of mental retardation, pp. 274–310 (Thomas, Springfield 1976).

3   Gooding, D.S.; Squires, K.S.; Starr, A.: Long latency event-related components of the auditory evoked potentials in dementia. Brain *101:* 635–648 (1978).

4   Gooding, D.S.; Starr, A.; Chippendale, T.; Squires, K.S.: Sequential changes in the P3 component of the auditory evoked potential in confusional states and dementing illness. Neurology, N.Y. *33:* 1215–1218 (1983).

5   Pfefferbaum, A.; Horwath, T.B.; Roth, T.B.; Kopell, B.S.: Event-related potentials changes in chronic alcoholics. Electroenceph. clin. Neurophysiol. *47:* 637–647 (1979).

6   Pfefferbaum, A.; Venegrat, B.G.; Ford, J.M.; Roth, W.T.; Koppel, B.S.: Clinical application of the P3 component of ERPs. II. Dementia, depression and schizophrenia. Electroenceph. clin. Neurophysiol. *59:* 104–124 (1984).

7   Squires, K.G.; Chippendale, T.J.; Wrege, K.W.; Gooding, D.W.; Starr, A.: Electrophysiological assessment of mental function in aging and dementia; in Poon, Aging in the 1980s, vol. 10, pp. 125–134 (Am. Physcological Association, Washington 1980).

8   Syndullko, K.; Hansch, E.C.; Cohen, S.N.; Pearce, J.W.; Goldberg, Z.; Montan, B.; Tourtellotte, W.W.; Potvin, A.R.: Long-latency event-regulated potentials in normal aging and dementia; in Courjon, Mauguiere, Revol, Clinical applications of evoked potentials in neurology. Adv. Neurol., vol. 32, pp. 279–285 (Raven Press, New York 1982).

9   Rizzo, P.A.; Albani, G.; Cicardi, C.; Spadaro, M.; Morocutti, C.: Effect of distraction on the contingent negative variation in presenile dementia and normal subjects. Neuropsychobiology *12:* 112–114 (1984).

10 Tecce, J.J.: Divided attention, ERPs, and aging: methodology and theory; in Karrer, Cohen, Tueting, Brain and information: event related potentials, pp. 497–502 (New York Academy of Sciences, New York 1984).

11 Tecce, J.J.; Cattanach, L.; Branconnier, R.J.: Absence of CNV rebound in Alzheimer's patients; in McCallum, Zappoli, Denoth, Cerebral psychophysiology: studies in

event-related potentials. Electroenceph. clin. Neurophysiol., suppl. 38, pp. 452–454 (1986).

12   Polich, J.; Ehlers, C.L.; Otis, S.; Mandell, A.J.; Bloom, F.E.: P300 latency reflects the degree of cognitive decline in dementing illness. Electroenceph. clin. Neurophysiol. *63:* 138–144 (1986).

13   Zappoli, R.; Arnetoli, G.; Paganini, M.; Versari, A.; Battaglia, A.; Grignani, A.; Porcù, S.: CNV activity and RT in patients with presenile idiopathic cognitive decline and presenile Alzheimer-type dementia: A preliminary report. Riv. It. Neurofisiol. Clin. *9:* 233–250 (1986).

14   Vaughan, H.G.: The relationship of brain activity to scalp recordings of event-related potentials; in Donchin, Lindsley, Averaged evoked potentials, pp. 45–94 (NASA, Washington 1969).

15   McCallum, W.C.; Curry, S.H.: The form and distribution of auditory evoked potentials and CNVs when stimuli and responses are lateralized; in Kornhüber, Deecke, Motivation, motor and sensory processes of the brain: electrical potentials, behaviour and clinical use. Prog. Brain Res. *54:* 767–775 (1980).

16   Hillyard, S.A.; Hink, R.F.; Schwent, V.L.; Pincton, T.W.: Electric signs of selective attention in the human brain. Science *172:* 1357–1360 (1973).

17   Hillyard, S.A.; Picton, T.W.; Regan, D.: Sensation, perception and attention: analysis using ERPs; in Callaway, Tueting, Koslow, Event-related potentials in man, pp. 223–321 (Academic Press, New York 1978).

18   Donald, W.D.; Young, M.J.: Habituation and rate decrements in the auditory vertex potential during selective listening; in Kornhüber, Deecke, Motivation, motor and sensory processes of the brain: electrical potentials, behaviour and clinical use. Prog. Brain Res. *54:* 331–336 (1980).

19   Gooding, D.S.; Squires, K.C.; Henderson, B.H.; Starr, A.: Age-related variations in evoked potentials to auditory stimuli in normal human subjects. Electroenceph. clin. Neurophysiol. *44:* 447–458 (1978).

20   Smith, D.B.D.; Thompson, L.W.; Michalewski, J.: Averaged evoked potential research in adult aging-status and prospects; in Poon, Aging in the 1980s, vol. 10, pp. 135–151 (Am. Psychological Ass., Washington 1980).

21   Dustman, R.E.; Beck, E.C.: The effect of maturation and aging on the waveform of visually evoked potentials. Electroenceph. clin. Neurophysiol. *26:* 2–11 (1969).

22   Drechsler, F.: Quantitative analysis of neurophysiological processes of the aging CNS. J. Neurol. *218:* 197–213 (1978).

23   Beck, E.C.; Swanson, C.; Dustman, R.F.: Long latency components of the visually evoked potential in man: effects on aging. Exp. Aging Res. *6:* 523–545 (1980).

24   Pfefferbaum, A.; Ford, J.M.; Roth, W.T.; Hopkins, W.F. III; Kopell, B.S.: Event-related potential changes in healthy aged females. Electroenceph. clin. Neurophysiol. *46:* 81–86 (1979).

25   Pfefferbaum, A.; Ford, J.M.; Roth, W.T.; Kopell, B.S.: Age differences in P3-reaction time association. Electroenceph. clin. Neurophysiol. *49:* 257–265 (1980).

26   Pfefferbaum, A.; Ford, J.M.; Roth, W.T.; Kopell, B.S.: Age-related changes in auditory event-related potentials. Electroenceph. clin. Neurophysiol. *49:* 266–276 (1980).

27   Brent, G.A.; Smith, D.B.D.; Michalewski, H.J.; Thompson, L.W.: Differences in the evoked potential in young and old subjects during habituation and dishabituation procedures. Psychophysiology *14:* 96–97 (1977).

28   Smith, D.B.D.; Michalewski, H.J.; Brent, G.A.; Thompson, L.W.: Auditory aver-
     aged evoked potentials and aging: factors of stimulus, task and topography. Biol.
     Psychol. *11:* 135–151 (1980).
29   Ford, J.M.; Hink, R.F.; Hopkins, W.F.; Roth, W.T.; Pfefferbaum, A.; Kopell, B.S.:
     Age effects on event-related potentials in a selective attention task. J. Geront. *34:*
     388–395 (1979).
30   Ford, J.M.; Roth, W.T.; Mohs, R.C.; Hopkins, W.F.; Kopell, B.S.: Event-related
     potentials recorded from young and old adults during a memory retrieval task. Elec-
     troenceph. clin. Neurophysiol. *47:* 450–459 (1979).
31   Walrath, L.C.; Hallman, L.E.: Habituation of the event-related potential in elderly
     and young subjects; in Karrer, Cohen, Tueting, Brain and information: event-related
     potentials, vol. 425, pp. 391–397 (New York Academy of Sciences 1984).
32   Klorman, R.; Thompson, L.; Ellingson, R.: Event-related brain potentials across the
     life span; in Callaway, Koslow, Event-related brain potentials in man, pp. 511–570
     (Plenum Press, New York 1978).
33   Michalewski, K.J.; Patterson, J.V.; Bowman, T.E.; Litzleman, D.K.; Thompson,
     L.W.: A comparison of the emitted late positive potential in older and young adults.
     J. Geront. *37:* 52–58 (1982).
34   Picton, T.W.; Stuss, D.T.; Champagne, S.C.; Nelson, R.F.: The effects of age on
     human event-related potentials. Psychophysiology *21:* 312–325 (1984).
35   Pfefferbaum, A.; Ford, J.M.; Wenegrat, B.G.; Roth, W.T.; Kopell, B.S.: Clinical
     application of the P3 component of event-related potentials. I. Normal aging. Elec-
     troenceph. clin. Neurophysiol. *59:* 85–103 (1984).
36   Allison, T.; Hurne, A.L.; Wood, C.C.; Goff, W.R.: Developmental and aging changes
     in somatosensory, auditory and visual evoked potentials. Electroenceph. clin. Neu-
     rophysiol. *58:* 14–24 (1984).
37   Barrett, G.; Neshige, R.; Shibasaki, H.: Human auditory and somatosensory event-
     related potentials: effects of response condition and age. Electroenceph. clin. Neu-
     rophysiol. *66:* 409–419 (1987).
38   Näätänen, R.; Simpson, M.; Loveless, N.E.: Stimulus deviance and evoked poten-
     tials. Biol. Psychol. *14:* 99–111 (1982).
39   Näätänen, R.; Picton, T.W.: N2 and automatic versus controlled processes; in
     McCallum, Zappoli, Denoth, Cerebral psychophysiology: studies in event-related
     potentials. Electroenceph. clin. Neurophysiol., suppl. 38, pp. 169–186 (1986).
40   Donchin, E.; Ritter, W.; McCallum, W.C.: Cognitive psychophysiology: the endog-
     enous components of the ERP; in Callaway, Tueting, Koslow, Event-related brain
     potentials in man. pp. 349–411 (Academic Press, New York 1978).
41   Donchin, E.: Event-related brain potentials: a tool in the study of human informa-
     tion on processing; in Begleiter, Evoked brain potentials and behaviour, vol. 2 (Ple-
     num Press, New York 1979).
42   Squires, N.K.; Squires, K.C.; Hillyard, S.A.: Two varieties of long-latency positive
     waves evoked by unpredictable auditory stimuli in man. Electroenceph. clin. Neu-
     rophysiol. *38:* 387–401 (1975).
43   Ford, J.M.; Duncan-Johnson, C.C.; Pfefferbaum, A.; Kopell, B.S.: Expectancy for
     events in old age: stimulus sequence effects of P300 and reaction time. J. Geront. *37:*
     696–704 (1982).
44   Brown, W.S.; Marsh, J.T.; La Rue, A.: Exponential electrophysiological aging: P3
     latency. Electroenceph. clin. Neurophysiol. *55:* 277–285 (1983).

45 Mullis, R.J.; Holcomb, P.J.; Diner, B.C.; Dykman, R.A.: The effect of aging on the P3 component of the visual event-related potential. Electroenceph. clin. Neurophysiol. *62:* 141–149 (1985).

46 Marsh, G.R.: Age differences in evoked potential correlates of a memory scanning process. Exp. Aging Res. *1:* 3–16 (1975).

47 Podlesny, J.A.; Dustman, R.E.: Age effects on heart rate, sustained potential, and P3 responses during reaction-time tasks. Neurobiol. Aging *3:* 1–9 (1982).

48 Tecce, J.J.,; Yrchik, D.A.; Meinbresse, D.; Dessonville, C.L.; Cole, J.O.: CNV rebound and aging. I. Attention functions; in Kornhüber, Deecke, Motivation, motor and sensory process of the brain: electrical potentials, behaviour and clinical use. Prog. Brain Res. *54:* 552–561 (1980).

49 Tecce, J.J.; Yrchik, D.A.; Meinbresse, D.; Dessonville, C.L.; Clifford, T.S.; Cole, O.J.: CNV rebound and aging. II. type A and B CNV shapes; in Kornhüber, Deecke, Motivation, motor and sensory processes of the brain: electrical potentials, behaviour and clinical use. Prog. Brain Res. *54:* 562–573 (1980).

50 Tecce, J.J.; Cattanach, L.; Yrchik, D.A.; Meinbresse, D.; Dessonville, C.L.: CNV rebound and aging. Electroenceph. clin. Neurophysiol. *54:* 175–186 (1982).

51 Friedman, D.; Vaughan, H.G.; Erlenmeyer-Kimling, L.: Event-related potentials components of the late positive complex in visual discrimination tasks. Electroenceph. clin. Neurophysiol. *45:* 319–330 (1978).

52 Kutas, M.; Hillyard, S.A.: Event-related brain potentials to semantically inappropriate and surprisingly large words. Biol. Psychol. *11:* 99–116 (1981).

53 McCallum, W.C.; Farmer, S.F.; Pocock, P.V.: The effects of physical and semantic incongruities on auditory event-related potentials. Electroenceph. clin. Neurophysiol. *59:* 477–488 (1984).

54 Harbin, T.J.; Marsh, G.R.; Harvey, M.T.: Differences in the late components of the event-related potential due to age and to semantic and non-semantic tasks. Electroenceph. clin. Neurophysiol. *59:* 489–496 (1984.

55 Rohrbaugh, J.W.; Syndulko, K.; Lindsley, D.B.: Cortical slow negative waves following non-paired stimuli: effects of task factors. Electroenceph. clin. Neurophysiol. *45:* 551–567 (1978).

56 Rohrbaugh, J.W.; Gaillard, A.W.K.: Sensory and motor aspect of the contingent negative variation; in Gaillard, Ritter, Tutorials in event-related potential research: endogenous components (Elsevier, Amsterdam 1983).

57 Ruchkin, D.S.; Sutton, S.; Stega, M.: Emitted P300 and slow wave event-related potentials in guessing and detection tasks. Electroencph. clin. Neurophysiol. *49:* 1–4 (1980).

58 Ruchkin, D.S.; Sutton, S.; Kietzman, M.L.; Silver, K.: Slow wave and P300 in signal detection. Electroenceph. clin. Neurophysiol. *50:* 35–47 (1980).

59 Zappoli, R.; Versari, A.; Paganini, M.; Arnetoli, G.; Roma, V.; Rossi, L.; Porcù, S.: Age differences in contingent negative variation (CNV) of healthy young adults and presenile subjects. Ital. J. Neurol. Sci. (in press).

60 Deecke, L.; Sched, P.; Kornhüber, H.H.: Distribution of readiness potential, premotion positivity, and motor potential of the human cerebral cortex preceding voluntary finger movements. Exp. Brain Res. *7:* 158–168 (1969).

61 Barrett, G.; Schibasaki, H.; Neshige, R.: Cortical potentials preceding voluntary movement: evidence for three periods of preparation in man. Electroenceph. clin. Neurophysiol. *63:* 327–339 (1986).

62 Deecke, L.; Englitz, H.G.; Shmitt, G.: Age dependence of the Bereitschaftspotential; in Otto, Multidisciplinary perspectives in event-related brain potential research, pp. 330–332 (US Environmental Protection Agency, Washington 1978).

63 Loveless, N.E.; Sandford, A.J.: Effects of age on the contingent negative variation and preparatory set in a reaction-time task. J. Geront. *29:* 52–63 (1974).

64 Loveless, N.E.: Aging effects in simple RT and voluntary movement paradigms; in Kornhüber, Deecke, Motivation, motor and sensory processes of the brain: electrical potentials, behaviour and clinical use. Prog. Brain Res. *54:* 547–551 (1980).

65 Walter, W.G.; Cooper, R.; Aldrige, V.J.; McCallum, W.C.; Winter, A.L.: Contingent negative variation: an electric sign of sensory motor association and expectancy in the human brain. Nature *203:* 380–384 (1964).

66 Tecce, J.J.; Cattanach, L.: Contingent negative variation; in Niedermeyer, Lopes da Silva, Electroencephalography: basic principles, clinical applications and related fields, pp. 543–562 (Urban & Schwarzenberg, Baltimore 1982).

67 Nakamura, M.; Fukui, Y.; Kadobayashi, I.; Kato, N.: A comparison of the CNV in young and old subjects: its relation to memory and personality. Electroenceph. clin. Neurophysiol. *46:* 337–344 (1979).

68 Tecce, J.J.: Contingent negative variation and attention functions in the aged; in Callaway, Tueting, Koslow, Event-related brain potentials in man, pp. 626–637 (Academic Press, New York 1978).

69 Marsh, G.R.; Thompson, L.W.: Effects of age on the contingent negative variation in a pitch discrimination task. J. Geront. *28:* 56–62 (1973).

70 Harkins, S.W.; Moss, S.F.; Thompson, L.W.; Nowlin, J.B.: Relationship between central and autonomic nervous system activity: correlates and psychomotor performance in elderly men. Exp. Aging Res. *5:* 409–423 (1976).

71 Schaie, J.P.; Syndulko, K.: Age differences in cortical activity associated with preparation to respond. Int. J. Behav. Devel. *1:* 255–261 (1978).

72 Michalewski, H.J.; Thompson, L.W.; Smith, D.B.D.; Patterson, J.V.; Bowman, T.E.; Litzelman, D.; Brent, G.: Age differences in the contingent negative variation (CNV): reduced frontal activity in the elderly. J. Geront. *35:* 542–549 (1980).

73 Thompson, L.W.; Nowlin, J.B.: Relation of increased attention to central and autonomic nervous system states; in Jarvik, Eisdorfer, Blum, Intellectual influences, pp. 107–124 (Springer, New York 1973).

74 Gaillard, A.W.K.: The CNV as an index of response preparation; in McCallum, Zappoli, Denoth, Cerebral psychophysiology: studies in event-related potentials. Electroenceph. clin. Neurophysiol., suppl. 38, pp. 196–206 (1986).

75 Roth, W.T.; Duncan, C.C.; Pfefferbaum, A.; Timsit-Berthier, M.: Applications of cognitive ERPs in psychiatric patients; in McCallum, Zappoli, Denoth, Cerebral psychophysiology: studies in event-related potentials. Electroenceph. clin. Neurophysiol., suppl. 38, pp. 419–438 (1986).

76 Kok, A.: The effect of warning stimulus novelty on the P300 and components of the contingent negative variation. Biol. Psychol. *6:* 219–233 (1978).

77 Albert, M.; Kaplan, E.: Organic implications of neurophysiological deficits in the elderly; in Poon, Fozard, Cermak, Arenberg, Thompson, New directions in memory and aging, pp. 403–432 (Erlbaum, Hillsdale 1980).

78 Scheibel, M.F.; Lindsay, R.D.; Tomiyasu, V.; Scheibel, A.B.: Progressive dendritic changes in aging human cortex. Expl Neurol. *47:* 392–403 (1975).

79   Brody, H.: Cell counts in cerebral cortex and brainstem; in Katzman, Terry, Bick, Alzheimer's disease, senile dementia and related disorders, pp. 345–351 (Raven Press, New York 1978).

80   Pearson, R.C.A.; Esiri, M.N.; Hiorns, R.W.; Wilcock, G.K.; Powell, T.P.S.: Anatomical correlates of the distribution of the pathological changes in the neocortex in Alzheimer disease. Proc. natn. Acad. Sci. USA *82:* 4531–4534 (1985).

81   Ford, J.M.; Pfefferbaum, A.: The utility of brain potentials in determining age-related changes in central nervous system and cognitive function; in Poon, Aging in the 1980s, vol. 10, pp. 67–134 (Am. Psychological Ass., Washington 1980).

82   Zappoli, R.; Armetoli, G.; Paganini, M.; Versari, A.; Battaglia, A.; Grighahi, A.; Sacchetti, G.: Contingent negative variation and reaction time in patients with presenile idiopathic cognitive decline and presenile Alzheimer-type dementia. Preliminary report on long-term nicergoline treatment. Neuropsychobiology *18:* 149–154 (1987).

Roberto Zappoli, MD, 2nd Neurological Institute, University of Florence, Viale Morgagni 85, I–50134 Florence (Italy)

Giannitrapani, Murri (eds.), The EEG of Mental Activities,
pp. 26–41 (Karger, Basel 1988)

EEG Differentiation between Alzheimer's and Non-Alzheimer's Dementias[1]

Duilio Giannitrapani, Joseph Collins

Veterans Administration Medical Center, Perry Point, Md., USA

If the EEG is to be used to distinguish Alzheimer's from non-Alzheimer's dementias, it first has to be capable of differentiating between normal and abnormal aging. In order to accomplish this, an analysis will be made first of EEG characteristics of normal aging and subsequently of EEG studies of Alzheimer's and non-Alzheimer's dementia. Then new data will be presented which demonstrate spectral analysis capabilities for this differentiation.

Normal Aging

Some of the earliest observations describing the features of the normal EEG in old age indicated the presence in this group of generalized slowing [37, 39]. This slowing consisted both of the absence of higher frequency dominant alpha and the proportionately greater presence of delta activity.

Given the observed increase in average frequency in the development of the individual from birth to adolescence [11], a recapitulation hypothesis in senescence with a progressive decrease of average frequency seemed to be appropriate. Since these studies were not longitudinal, however, this progressive decrease in average frequency had not been observed directly but was inferred from the statistics. Early findings attesting to the remarkable stability of the frequency of dominant alpha in the aged population [5] were discounted in favor of the recapitulation hypothesis.

[1] This study was supported in part by the Veterans Administration Medical Center, Perry Point, Md., USA.

More recently, however, there has been increasing evidence that EEG slowing is not necessarily progressive with age [16, 17, 22, 54]. Even the increase in theta activity with age is being questioned, beginning with the research of Mundy-Castle [35] who found a greater percentage of theta in normal adults than in normal seniles having a mean age of 75 years.

Another EEG feature characteristic of senescence consists of focal abnormalities primarily in the temporal and anterior temporal areas on the left side. Since these focal abnormalities have been observed in subjects with and without brain pathology [36, 38], the clinical significance of these perhaps incorrectly termed abnormalities is not understood. Focal abnormalities in the aged, therefore, are regarded as being clinically silent without, at present, pathological significance.

An additional EEG feature characteristic of senescence consists of an observed increase in beta activity [13]. Greenblatt's early observations include peaking of beta activity in the 45- to 55-year-old group. Since his study dealt primarily with neuropsychiatric patients, it appeared that this feature was characteristic of psychopathology. Later observations, however [38], found a similar distribution of beta activity in normal aging, lending support to the notion that the presence of fast activity in the EEG of the aged is not symptomatic of pathology [36].

Against this background of the current knowledge of EEG characteristics in normal senescence, the EEG features characteristic of patients with various types of dementia will be compared.

The EEG in Dementia

Traditional clinical EEG correlates in senile dementia of the Alzheimer's type (SDAT) consist of dominant alpha slowing, diffuse slowing and disorganization [26, 28, 50–52] while intermittent lateralized slow waves or slow waves alternating between the hemispheres suggest artery disease [34]. Similarly, multi-infarct dementia patients differ significantly from SDAT patients only in asymmetric findings [29, 47]. On the other hand, Pick disease patients having psychometric defects comparable to SDAT patients include EEG records void of abnormalities [20].

Central to this investigation is determining whether the severity of dementia of the Alzheimer's type can be measured by EEG parameters. Gordon and Sim [12] found in early Alzheimer's a reduction or absence of alpha while later they found an increase in theta and delta activity. The latter observation was made also by Ingvar et al. [19] and Prinz et al. [42].

Kaszniak et al. [23], studying a sample of patients with suspected dementia (selected for absence of focal neurologic or other organic disease), found negative correlations between EEG slowing or cortical atrophy and a series of psychological measures which required a cognitive response on the part of the patient.

Merskey et al. [33] used a delta and a dysrhythmia score singly and in combination. They found that the EEG dysrhythmia correlated best in less severe degrees of dementia. Correlations were weaker with delta activity in a sample which included also the most severe degree of dementia. Their best correlation was obtained between the combined Z-scores for the physical measures (which included a CT-derived ventricular enlargement score) and the Z-scores for the psychological measures (which included the Extended Scale for Dementia and the London Psychogeriatric Rating Scale).

Finally, Soininen et al. [48], studying a group of moderate to severe dementia, found that the highest discriminant function coefficient among the EEG variables was for dominant occipital rhythm followed by diffuse slowing.

The above analyses suggest that differentiation between Alzheimer's and non-Alzheimer's dementia is possible through the EEG. The nature of the difference is in terms of greater severity of EEG abnormalities in SDAT. Given the problems in measuring the severity of the dementia, a method for quantifying EEG slowing and frequency of dominant alpha was needed which would offer greater reliability than visual inspection. Following is the analysis of EEG spectral analysis findings.

Frequency Analysis Studies

Matoušek et al. [30] studied the EEG characteristics in an age range from 17 to 64 years from 2 frontal and 2 temporo-parietal derivations. They found several significant relationships between age and 6 broad EEG frequency bands. These findings, even though significant, were characterized by such great interindividual scatter as to render predictive validity impossible. Notable, however, is the observed negative relationship between both delta and theta activity and age. This observation appears at first sight to contradict (at least for this relatively younger age group) the previously mentioned observed increase of slow activity with age. It suggests that the presence of slow activity in senescence is a result of a different process than that present prior to the sixth decade, and it supports the above mentioned evidence that even in the older individual EEG slowing is not progressive with age.

Roubíček [45], with a broad-band frequency analysis of the EEG and an age range between 60 and 90, reaffirmed the increase of slow waves with age and a shift of dominant frequency from 9 to 7 Hz.

Liberson and Fried [27], performing a narrow-band frequency analysis of 75- to 92-year-olds, found an association between confusion and the absence of significant 8 Hz activity (or faster) in the parieto-occipital regions.

Stigsby et al. [49], with an EEG narrow-band frequency analysis, studied 9 Alzheimer's patients and 4 patients with Pick disease. The Alzheimer's patients showed diffuse slowing in all regions, increased delta and theta activity, and decreased alpha and beta activity. In the Pick patients alpha activity was preserved, and the delta and theta increase was not as pronounced as that in the Alzheimer's. Even though Pick patients are usually considered to have a relatively intact EEG (even in advanced stages of dementia), the 2 groups were not matched for dementia. Definitive conclusions, therefore, cannot be drawn from the differences observed in their study.

A longitudinal study of Alzheimer's patients having mild dementia was made by Coben et al. [4] with narrow-band frequency analysis. As compared to a control group, a significant increase was found for theta activity and a decrease in beta.

Berg et al. [2] compared a sample of mild SDAT patients with normal controls. They found that the SDAT group had decreased beta power and increased theta power with no difference in alpha and delta power.

Visser et al. [56] studied a group of SDAT patients which appeared to be in the mild to moderate range. They compared this group with a group of normal subjects and a group with nonorganic behavioral disorders. The EEG power density spectrum of the SDAT patients showed a decreased mean frequency of the total spectrum as well as decreased mean frequency of the theta band. They also found an increase in the relative power in delta and theta bands and a decrease in relative power in alpha and beta bands.

Finally, Penttila et al. [40] performed narrow-band frequency analysis on patients in different stages of Alzheimer's disease. While in mild SDAT relative theta power increased and the mean frequency decreased, in advanced SDAT occipital peak frequency slowing and increase of relative power of the delta band were observed.

In summary, the preponderance of the evidence from both traditional clinical EEG and EEG spectral analysis is that in dementia there is a slowing of the dominant frequency, an increase in theta and delta activity and in mild dementia a possible increase in beta activity. Differentiation between Alzheimer's dementia and other forms of dementia has not been adequately studied.

Previous research by the present investigator [10] suggested that while an increase in slow activity should be expected with a decrease of intellectual functions, an increase in fast activity was related to a facility for solving comprehension and arithmetic problems. In senescence it may consist of a by-product of a coping mechanism to counteract the decrease in intellectual functions. In the later stages of the dementia, therefore, an increase in fast activity should not occur.

The Dementia Scale

Crucial for determining the existence of relationships between EEG parameters and the severity of the dementia is the development of a reliable dementia scale. The literature is replete with dementia and mental status examinations, most being void of norms and of any attempt at validation, and the scores are added without any attempt to satisfy equal interval requirements. Some are extensions of intelligence tests [57]. Others require some kind of behavioral response [1, 21]. The remainder are rating scales [46, 55]. Most of the tests do not penetrate the floor of the severe dementia category [7, 8, 14, 18, 24, 25, 41].

The clinical definition of severe dementia consists of a major loss of abstraction that prevents the patient from living in the community even in a sheltered environment. Language functions can be intact to a considerable extent. More extreme forms of dementia usually present different medical problems which clinically determine the primary treatment modality of the patient, e.g. nutrition, metabolism, preservation of vital signs.

The few scales that do penetrate the severe dementia category offer very little dimensionality in the lower range [3, 15, 31, 32, 43, 53, 58, 60] and do not have a clear hierarchy of responses. The overall deficit is not

Table I. The 11-point dementia scale

Scores	Criteria
0	No impairment
1	Anomia only
2	Moderate memory impairment and anomia
3	Abstractions still present but severe memory impairment
4	Speech still coherent, concrete and limited to social stereotypes
5	Occasionally capable of coherent response with sentence
6	Speech still present, mostly jargon
7	Minimally vocally responsive to verbal or visual stimuli
8	Responds to name with eyes only
9	Minimally responsive to verbal or visual stimuli with eyes only
10	Nonresponsive

immediately apparent. It has to be inferred from the specific deficits and then derived from an analysis of the responses, a matter which adds to the unreliability of the scoring especially when compounded with the problems surrounding the equal interval issue.

These shortcomings are difficult to avoid because in mental testing item difficulty is arrived at strictly on a pragmatic basis, and the theoretical framework is superimposed only to fit the data. Even though this may be the best available method for constructing mental tests in the normal range, the derived tenets have little utility when applying this hierarchy to the responses obtained from subjects suffering from a myriad of brain disorders. Our knowledge of the manner in which language and thinking are performed by the brain is woefully inadequate for the determination of a precise hierarchy of responses which is neurophysiologically meaningful.

For the present investigation an 11-point cognitive scale was developed, based upon developmental theory [59]. In the search for EEG parameters symptomatic of dementia, the extreme cases needed to be studied. In this investigation it was deemed necessary to carry out the concept of dementia to its extreme, the semicomatose state usually regarded as a problem of consciousness rather than as dementia per se.

To provide a simple instrument able to rank patients on a broad spectrum of deficits, the dementia scale developed (table I) ranks impairments in naming, memory, abstraction, speech, voice, orientation and perception. Please note that scoring on this scale is valid only when the deficits observed are due to an implied dementia process and not due to peripheral processes which would prevent the response.

Method

Three groups of male subjects were studied: (1) 16 patients with a diagnosis of severe Alzheimer's disease; (2) 16 patients with various diagnoses of dementia exclusive of Alzheimer's (primarily vascular or metabolic in origin), and (3) 10 normal control subjects. All subjects of the 2 patient groups were inpatients at the Veterans Administration Medical Center, Perry Point, Md. The 3 groups were matched for age: Alzheimer's age range 54–81 (mean = 67.4), non-Alzheimer's dementia age range 45–89 (mean = 66.6) and control age range 48–84 (mean = 63.5). In addition, the 2 groups of patients were matched for dementia using the 11-point dementia scale developed for this study (table I). This developmental behavioral rating scale is expanded in the severe range of the scale. The Alzheimer's patients range from 3 to 9 on this scale (mean = 5.4), and the non-Alzheimer's dementia patients ranged from 2 to 9 (mean = 5.0). All patients had the study described to them prior to participation, and they or their guardians signed an informed consent.

Patients were under a variety of medications which were not controlled for the purpose of this experiment. Levels and types of medications were grossly comparable for the 2 groups of patients. Three of the subjects of the normal control group were taking psychotropic medication.

A traditional EEG examination with 12 monopolar derivations (linked ears as reference) according to the 10–20 system was administered: F_3, F_4, F_7, F_8, T_3, T_4, C_3, C_4, P_3, P_4, O_1, O_2. Low frequency filter setting was at 0.3 Hz in order to provide a time constant and yet minimize the low frequency distortion introduced by the filters. High frequency filter setting was placed at 70 Hz.

Spectral analysis of the EEG was performed on a Rockland Spectrum Analyzer during an awake-resting condition, and the power spectral values were recorded on an X-Y plotter for 2 consecutive 8-second periods which were averaged separately for each of the 12 brain areas. In the event that movement artifacts occurred during these 16 s, they were discarded and an additional 16-second segment was recorded and analyzed. The 400-point spectrum was frequency averaged in order to obtain 18 2-Hz-wide frequency bands from 0 to 36 Hz. These 18 spectral values were log transformed and then averaged over the 12 brain areas. They will be referred to hereafter as power scores. During the recording, patients were closely monitored for the occurrence of drowsiness which was prevented by alerting the patient whenever necessary, i.e. when flattening or slowing was observed in the raw EEG as compared with the initial awake-resting levels. Recording was obtained while patient had eyes closed except in the cases of most severe dementia in which the patient did not understand the directions and/or would not cooperate. In those cases it was observed that the characteristic EEG differences between the eyes-open and eyes-closed conditions did not occur.

The variables used in this study were the dementia scores and the power scores for the mean of the 12 brain areas for each of the 18 2-Hz-wide frequency bands. Analyses of

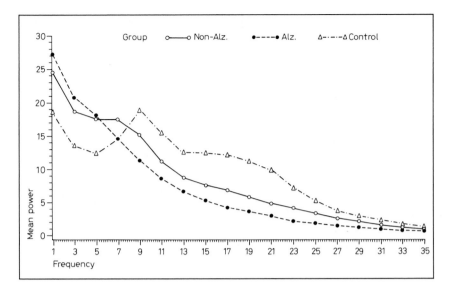

Fig. 1. Twelve brain areas' mean $\log_{10}$ power scores vs 18 frequency bands (2-Hz wide, 0–36 Hz) for 3 groups: Alzheimer's dementia patients (n = 16), non-Alzheimer's dementia patients (n = 16) and normal controls (n = 10).

variance were used to detect differences in power scores at the various frequencies between the Alzheimer's group, the non-Alzheimer's demented group and the controls. When these analyses were statistically significant, Bonferroni t-tests were used to determine which groups were statistically different from each other. The final analysis performed was a stepwise discriminant analysis to determine which of the study variables best discriminated between the Alzheimer's group and the non-Alzheimer's demented group.

Results

The means of the power scores for the 3 groups are plotted in figure 1. It shows that for the 1-, 3- and 5-Hz frequency bands the control subjects have significantly lower power scores than those in either the Alzheimer's or the non-Alzheimer's dementia groups and have significantly higher power scores than the 2 dementia groups at the 11-, 13-, 15-, 17-, 19-, 21- and 23-Hz frequency bands. At the 9-, 25- and 27-Hz frequency bands the control group also has significantly higher power scores than the Alzheimer's group. The crossover from significantly lower power scores to significantly higher power scores occurs at the 7-Hz frequency band. The only statistically different power score between the Alzheimer's and non-Alzheimer's dementia groups is a significantly higher 9-Hz frequency band score for the non-Alzheimer's dementia patients.

The role of the different frequency bands in distinguishing the dementias was studied further through discriminant function analysis. Since the number of variables was relatively large in comparison to the number of subjects, the significance of the results of the discriminant analysis should be reviewed with caution and should not be considered to be per se of statistical significance. The variables studied consisted of means of the 12 brain areas for each of the 18 frequency bands as well as the dementia scores. The significant variables were mean of 9 Hz, mean of 1 Hz and the dementia score in order of decreasing importance. The resulting discrimination between the Alzheimer's and non-Alzheimer's groups misclassifies one Alzheimer's patient and 4 non-Alzheimer's patients.

Discussion

The control group retains a previously observed alpha peak at 9 Hz [45]. This represents a slowing from a mean dominant frequency of 11 Hz observed in younger ages. Of particular interest in this normal group is the hump of activities in the 15- to 21-Hz frequencies. The power of this activity is significantly decreased in the non-Alzheimer's dementia group and is decreased further in the Alzheimer's patients.

Earlier investigators had observed an increase in fast activity with increase in age. This increase was not positively correlated with dementia but rather seemed to relate to intact functions. The present investigator [9] postulated that the amplitude of low beta activity could represent the presence of a mechanism for scanning for structure on the basis of the observation that an increase in this activity occurred in the presence of unstructured stimuli or stimuli that required structuring on the part of the subject. Later observations in a young adolescent group [10] indicated that the amplitude of low beta activity (among other frequencies) correlated positively with the capacity for performance on the Comprehension, the Arithmetic (fig. 2), Picture Arrangement (fig. 3) and Block Design subtests of the WISC (Wechsler Intelligence Scale for Children). All of these subtests require a structuring effort on the part of the subject.

		Frequency bands															
		1	3	5	7	9	11	13	15	17	19	21	23	25	27	29	31
Prefrontal	left																
	right																
Lat. frontal	left							●									
	right							•									
Frontal	left							●	•				•	•			
	right							●	•	•							
Central	left							●	•	•							
	right							●		•							
Temporal	left							●	•	•							
	right							●	•								
Post-temporal	left							•		●				•			
	right																
Parietal	left							•		•				•			
	right							•		•							
Occipital	left									•				•	•		
	right									•				•			

• Rho with p < 0.05 (0.26–0.34); ● rho with p < 0.01 (0.35–0.42); ● rho with p < 0.001 (0.43–0.48); ■ rho with p < 0.0001 (> 0.48).
A minus (–) preceding the dot indicates a negative rho.

2

		Frequency bands															
		1	3	5	7	9	11	13	15	17	19	21	23	25	27	29	31
Prefrontal	left																
	right																
Lat. frontal	left			–•													
	right			–•	–•												
Frontal	left																
	right									•							
Central	left							•	●	●							•
	right								•	•							
Temporal	left																
	right								•		•						
Post-temporal	left							•									
	right									•							
Parietal	left								•	•							•
	right								•	●	•						
Occipital	left							•		●	•		•	•			
	right									•		•					

• Rho with p < 0.05 (0.26–0.34); ● rho with p < 0.01 (0.35–0.42); ● rho with p < 0.001 (0.43–0.48); ■ rho with p < 0.0001 (> 0.48).
A minus (–) preceding the dot indicates a negative rho.

3

Fig. 2. Matrix of significant correlations between EEG power scores (16 frequency bands, 2-Hz wide, 0–32 Hz) and the weighted scores of the WISC Arithmetic subtest (n = 56; 11- to 13-year-olds). Notice the strong correlations in the 13-Hz band which are common to most (primarily Verbal) subtests.

Fig. 3. Matrix of significant correlations between EEG power scores (16 frequency bands, 2-Hz wide, 0–32 Hz) and the weighted scores of the WISC Picture Arrangement subtest (n = 56; 11- to 13-year-olds).

		Frequency bands															
		1	3	5	7	9	11	13	15	17	19	21	23	25	27	29	31
Prefrontal	left																
	right							•									
Lat. frontal	left				•		•	■	•				•				
	right						•	•	•								
Frontal	left			•	•		•	■	●	•	•	●	●	•			
	right			•		•	•	■	•	●	●	●	●				
Central	left	●	●				•	■	●	●			•				
	right	•					•	■	●	●			●		•		
Temporal	left	●					•	●	●	•	•						
	right						•	●	●								
Post-temporal	left			•			•	●	•	●							
	right									•							
Parietal	left		•				•	●	●	●			•				
	right	•	•				•	●	●	•							
Occipital	left																
	right		●														

• Rho with p < 0.05 (0.26–0.34); ● rho with p < 0.01 (0.35–0.42); ● rho with p < 0.001 (0.43–0.48); ■ rho with p < 0.0001 (> 0.48). A minus (–) preceding the dot indicates a negative rho.

Fig. 4. Matrix of significant correlations between the same EEG power scores of figures 2 and 3 and the factor loadings of Davis' factor F, weighted on the WISC Comprehension and Arithmetic subtests.

Of the several factor analytic studies of the WISC, Davis [6] isolated a factor loaded on the Arithmetic and Comprehension subtests which, when applied to Giannitrapani's data (fig. 4), best focuses on the role of low beta activity in cognitive functions.

These 2 hypotheses, the first suggesting scanning for structure and the second suggesting conceptual ability as a correlate to the amplitude of low beta activity, are not mutually exclusive. They are consistent with the findings of the present experiment which show a significantly higher level of low beta activity in the normal control group and no significant differences in this activity between the 2 demented groups.

The Non-Alzheimer's Dementia Group

The non-Alzheimer's dementia group shows an absence of dominant peaks but a semblance of dominant activity on or about 7 Hz. This indicates that dominant activity is less prominent and, in general, slower than in the normal control group. The non-Alzheimer's dementia group also shows significantly more slow activity and significantly less fast activity (low beta) than the normal control group.

These findings indicate that in the case of non-Alzheimer's dementia it is meaningful to speak of slowing of dominant activity because the rhythmical organization of dominant activity is by and large retained in these patients. This is to be contrasted with the absence of dominant rhythmical activity to be discussed later in the context of Alzheimer's dementia.

The Alzheimer's Group

The Alzheimer's group is conspicuous for having a spectrum void of features. It consists of an exponential curve decreasing in power with increasing frequency. While all of the Alzheimer's patients followed this pattern, there were only 4 subjects of the non-Alzheimer's dementia group who had this pattern, and 2 of these were extremely demented (dementia scores = 9). Possibilities for the presence of the Alzheimer's pattern in the more severely demented of the non-Alzheimer's group include (1) misclassification or (2) that dementia, whatever its cause, eventually will reach a point in which the portion of the structural changes directly responsible for the dementia in both the non-Alzheimer's dementia process and the Alzheimer's process are indistinguishable.

The crossover for the Alzheimer's and control power curves occurs at 7 Hz while the non-Alzheimer's dementia group shows an increase at that frequency. Given the Alzheimer's-normal group crossover, the shape of the spectrum in the non-Alzheimer's group gives the 7-Hz activity a particular meaning. There is a slowing of dominant activity rather than an increase in slow activity unrelated to the rhythmicity of dominant activity. The latter is evident in the higher power of the lower frequency bands in the spectra of the Alzheimer's patients.

The independence of delta and theta power from the slowing of dominant activity has been observed previously [30]. In other words, the non-Alzheimer's dementia group retains a capacity for rhythmicity with a dominant frequency band, even though it is slower than for the normals. The Alzheimer's group shows no such organization of rhythmic activity. This points, perhaps, to the basic difference between the structural changes prevalent in Alzheimer's disease as compared with the changes consequent to vascular or metabolic diseases and may account for the historically low correlation between histologic alterations and intellectual impairment [3, 44].

Various EEG features associated with Alzheimer's disease, including an increase in theta and delta and a decrease in the frequency of dominant activity, have been observed by investigators using traditional visual inspection of the EEG [26, 34].

The asymptotic spectral curve of the severe Alzheimer's patient has not been observed previously. This might be due to the fact that this type of curve might not be present in the early stages of Alzheimer's dementia. Furthermore, spectral analysis studies concentrated on the utilization of relationships or ratios among traditional broadband EEG frequencies, a method which would not make apparent the overall shape of the curve. Traditional broadband EEG frequencies would also mask the differential between the Alzheimer's and non-Alzheimer's patients observed in this study. A decrease in fast activity and an increase in slow activity can be used to characterize both the asymptotic spectrum (Alzheimer's) and the decrease in amount of fast activity as well as the decrease in frequency of dominant activity (non-Alzheimer's).

The discriminant function analysis findings provide further evidence for isolating the 1-Hz band (0–2 Hz) from the remainder of delta and theta activity. The significant frequency bands are 1 and 9 Hz. The discriminant analysis coefficients show, basically, an inverse relationship between these 2 frequency bands in differentiating between Alzheimer's and non-Alzheimer's patients.

In this study, we have shown that there are differences between Alzheimer's patients, non-Alzheimer's dementia patients and controls. We have found what could be a pathognomonic feature of severe Alzheimer's dementia, i.e. a power spectral curve having a maximum at 1 Hz and an exponential asymptotic curve characterized by decreasing power with increasing frequency without additional features or a remnant of dominant activity. In addition, we have demonstrated that the decrease in the frequency of dominant activity is significant in identifying dementia of the non-Alzheimer's type and that increase in beta activity is characteristic of normal senescence.

References

1   Benton, A.L.: A visual retention test for clinical use. Archs Neurol. Psychiat., Chicago 54: 212–216 (1945).
2   Berg, L.; Danziger, W.L.; Storandt, M.; Coben, L.A.; Gado, M.; Hughes, C.P.; Knesevich, J.W.; Botwinick, J.: Predictive features in mild senile dementia of the Alzheimer type. Neurology, Cleveland 34: 563–569 (1984).

3   Blessed, G.; Tomlinson, B.E.; Roth, M.: The association between quantitative mea-
    sures of dementia and of senile change in the cerebral grey matter of elderly subjects.
    Br. J. Psychiat. *114:* 797–811 (1968).
4   Coben, L.A.; Danziger, W.L.; Berg, L.: Frequency analysis of the resting awake EEG
    in mild senile dementia of Alzheimer type. Electroenceph. clin. Neurophysiol. *55:*
    372–380 (1983).
5   Davis, P.A.: The electroencephalogram in old age. Dis. nerv. Syst. *2:* 77 (1941).
6   Davis, P.C.: A factor analysis of the Wechsler-Bellevue Scale. Educ. Psychol.
    Measmt *16:* 127–146 (1956).
7   Fishback, D.B.: Mental status questionnaire for organic brain syndrome, with a new
    visual counting test. J. Am. Geriat. Soc. *25:* 167–170 (1977).
8   Folstein, M.F.; Folstein, S.E.; McHugh, P.R.: Mini-mental state. J. psychiat. Res. *12:*
    189–198 (1975).
9   Giannitrapani, D.: Scanning mechanisms and the EEG. Electroenceph. clin. Neuro-
    physiol. *30:* 139–146 (1971).
10 Giannitrapani, D.: The electrophysiology of intellectual functions (Karger, Basel
    1985).
11 Gibbs, F.A.; Knott, J.R.: Growth of the electrical activity of the cortex. Electroen-
    ceph. clin. Neurophysiol. *1:* 223–229 (1949).
12 Gordon, E.B.; Sim, M.: The EEG in presenile dementia. J. Neurol. Neurosurg. Psy-
    chiat. *30:* 285–291 (1967).
13 Greenblatt, M.: Age and electroencephalographic abnormality in neuropsychiatric
    patients, a study of 1593 cases. Am. J. Psychiat. *101:* 82–90 (1944).
14 Gurland, B.J.: The assessment of the mental health status of older adults; in Birren,
    Sloane, Handbook of mental health and aging, pp. 671–700 (Prentice-Hall, New
    York 1980).
15 Gurland, B.J.; Dean, L.L.; Copeland, J.; Gurland, R.; Golden, R.: Criteria for the
    diagnosis of dementia in the community elderly. Gerontologist *22:* 180–186
    (1982).
16 Hubbard, O.; Sunde, D.; Goldensohn, E.S.: The EEG in centenarians. Electroen-
    ceph. clin. Neurophysiol. *40:* 407–417 (1976).
17 Hughes, J.R.; Cayaffa, J.J.: The EEG in patients at different ages without organic
    cerebral disease. Electroenceph. clin. Neurophysiol. *42:* 776–784 (1977).
18 Hughes, C.P.; Berg, L.; Danziger, W.L.; Coben, L.A.; Martin, R.L.: A new clinical
    scale for the staging of dementia. Br. J. Psychiat. *140:* 566–572 (1982).
19 Ingvar, D.H.; Johannesson, G.; Stigsby, B.: Regional cerebral blood flow and EEG in
    organic dementia, a brief review. Rev. Electroencéphalogr. Neurophysiol. clin. *10:*
    270–275 (1980).
20 Johannesson, G.; Hagberg, B.; Gustafson, L.; Ingvar, D.H.: EEG and cognitive
    impairment in presenile dementia. Acta neur. scand. *59:* 225–240 (1979).
21 Kahn, R.L.; Goldfarb, A.I.; Pollack, M.; Peck, A.: Brief objective measures for the
    determination of mental status in the aged. Am. J. Psychiat. *117:* 326–328 (1960).
22 Katz, R.I.; Horowitz, G.R.: Electroencephalogram in the septuagenarian: studies in
    a normal geriatric population. J. Am. Geriat. Soc. *30:* 273–275 (1982).
23 Kaszniak, A.W.; Garron, D.C.; Fox, J.H.; Bergen, D.; Huckman, M.: Cerebral atro-
    phy, EEG slowing, age, education, and cognitive functioning in suspected dementia.
    Neurology, Minneap. *29:* 1273–1279 (1979).

24 Lawton, M.P.: The functional assessment of elderly people. J. Am. Geriat. Soc. *19:* 465–481 (1971).
25 Lawton, M.P.; Moss, M.; Fulcomer, M.; Kleban, M.H.: A research and service oriented multilevel assessment instrument. J. Geront. *37:* 91–99 (1982).
26 Letemendia, F.; Pampiglione, G.: Clinical and electroencephalographic observations in Alzheimer's disease. J. Neurol. Neurosurg. Psychiat. *21:* 167–172 (1958).
27 Liberson, W.T.; Fried, P.: EEG power spectrum and confusion in the elderly. Electromyogr. clin. Neurophysiol. *21:* 353–367 (1981).
28 Liddell, D.W.: Investigations of EEG findings in presenile dementia. J. Neurol. Neurosurg. Psychiat. *21:* 173–176 (1958).
29 Logar, C.; Enge, S.; Ladurner, G.; Bertha, G.; Schneider, G.; Lechner, H.: Das EEG bei Multiinfarkten mit und ohne intellektuellen Abbau. Z. EEG-EMG *14:* 204–208 (1983).
30 Matoušek, M.; Volavka, J.; Roubíček, J.; Roth, Z.: EEG frequency analysis related to age in normal adults. Electroenceph. clin. Neurophysiol. *23:* 162–167 (1967).
31 Mattis, S.: Mental status examination for organic mental syndrome in the elderly patient; in Bellak, Karasu, Geriatric psychiatry, pp. 77–121 (Grune & Stratton, New York 1976).
32 Meer, B.; Baker, J.A.: The Stockton geriatric rating scale. J. Geront. *21:* 392–403 (1966).
33 Mersky, H.; Ball, M.J.; Blume, W.T.; Fox, A.J.; Fox, H.; Hersch, E.L.; Kral, V.A.; Palmer, R.B.: Relationships between psychological measurements and cerebral organic changes in Alzheimer's disease. Can. J. neurol. Sci. *7:* 45–49 (1980).
34 Müller, H.F.: The electroencephalogram in senile dementia; in Nandy, Senile dementia: a biomedical approach, pp. 237–250 (Elsevier, North-Holland Biomedical Press, Amsterdam 1978).
35 Mundy-Castle, A.C.: Theta and beta rhythm in the electroencephalograms of normal adults. Electroenceph. clin. Neurophysiol. *3:* 477–486 (1951).
36 Niedermeyer, E.: EEG and old age; in Niedermeyer; Lopes da Silva, Electroencephalography: basic principles and clinical practice, pp. 255–261 (Urban & Schwarzenberg, Baltimore 1982).
37 Obrist, W.D.: The electroencephalogram of normal aged adults. Electroenceph. clin. Neurophysiol. *6:* 235–244 (1954).
38 Obrist, W.D.: Problems of aging; in Remond, Handbook of electroencephalography and clinical neurophysiology, vol. 6A, pp. 275–292 (Elsevier, Amsterdam 1976).
39 Otomo, E.: Electroencephalography in old age: dominant alpha pattern. Electroenceph. clin. Neurophysiol. *21:* 489–491 (1966).
40 Penttila, M.; Partanen, J.V.; Soininen, H.; Riekkinen, P.J.: Quantitative analysis of occipital EEG in different stages of Alzheimer's disease. Electroenceph. clin. Neurophysiol. *60:* 1–6 (1985).
41 Pfeiffer, E.: A short portable mental status questionnaire for the assessment of organic brain deficit in elderly patients. J. Am. Geriat. Soc. *23:* 433–441 (1975).
42 Prinz, P.N.; Vitaliano, P.P.; Vitiello, M.V.; Bokan, J.; Raskind, M.; Peskind, E.; Gerber, C.: Sleep, EEG and mental function changes in senile dementia of the Alzheimer's type. Neurobiol. Aging *3:* 361–370 (1982).
43 Reisberg, B.; Ferris, S.H.; Crook, T.: Signs, symptoms and course of age-associated cognitive decline; in Corkin et al., Alzheimer's disease: a review of progress. Aging, vol. 19, pp. 177–181 (Raven Press, New York 1982).

44 Rothschild, D.: Pathologic changes in senile psychoses and their psychobiologic significance. Am. J. Psychiat. *93:* 757–788 (1937).
45 Roubíček, J.: The electroencephalogram in the middle-aged and the elderly. J. Am. Geriat. Soc. *25:* 145–152 (1977).
46 Salzman, C.; Kochansky, G.E.; Shader, R.I.: Rating scales for geriatric psychopharmacology – a review. Psychopharmacol. Bull. *8:* 3–50 (1972).
47 Soininen, H.; Partanen, V.J.; Helkala, E.-L.; Riekkinen, P.J.: EEG findings in senile dementia and normal aging. Acta neurol. scand. *65:* 59–70 (1982).
48 Soininen, H.; Partanen, J.V.; Puranen, M.; Riekkinen, P.J.: EEG and computed tomography in the investigation of patients with senile dementia. J. Neurol. Neurosurg. Psychiat. *45:* 711–714 (1982).
49 Stigsby, B.; Johannesson, G.; Ingvar, D.H.: Regional EEG analysis and regional cerebral blood flow in Alzheimer's and Pick's diseases. Electroenceph. clin. Neurophysiol. *51:* 537–547 (1981).
50 Striano, S.; Vacca, G.; Bilo, L.; Meo, R.: The electroencephalogram in dementia, differential diagnostic value in Alzheimer's disease, senile dementia and multiinfarct dementia. Acta neurol., Napoli *36:* 727–734 (1981).
51 Sulkava, R.: Alzheimer's disease and senile dementia of Alzheimer type, a comparative study. Acta neurol. scand. *65:* 636–650 (1982).
52 Swain, J.M.: Electroencephalographic abnormalities in presenile atrophy. Neurology, Minneap. *9:* 722–727 (1959).
53 Taylor, H.G.; Bloom, L.M.: Cross-validation and methodological extension of the Stockton geriatric rating scale. J. Geront. *29:* 190–193 (1974).
54 Torres, F.; Faoro, A.; Loewenson, R.; Johnson, E.: The electroencephalogram of elderly subjects revisited. Electroenceph. clin. Neurophysiol. *56:* 391–398 (1983).
55 Trier, T.R.: A study of change among elderly psychiatric inpatients during their first year of hospitalization. J. Geront. *23:* 354–362 (1968).
56 Visser, S.L.; Van Tilburg, W.; Hooijer, C.; Jonker, C.; De Rijke, W.: Visual evoked potentials (VEPs) in senile dementia (Alzheimer type) and in non-organic behavioural disorders in the elderly; comparison with EEG parameters. Electroenceph. clin. Neurophysiol. *60:* 115–121 (1985).
57 Wechsler, D.: A standardized memory scale for clinical use. J. Psychol. *19:* 87–95 (1945).
58 Wells, F.L.; Ruesch, J.: Mental examiner's handbook (Psychological Corporation, New York 1945).
59 Werner, H.: Comparative psychology of mental development (International Universities Press, New York 1957).
60 Zemcov, A.; Barclay, L.L.; Brush, D.; Blass, J.P.: Computerized data base for evaluation and follow-up of demented outpatients. J. Am. Geriat. Soc. *32:* 801–842 (1984).

Duilio Giannitrapani, PhD, Veterans Administration Medical Center, PO Box 193, Perry Point, MD 21902 (USA)

Giannitrapani, Murri (eds.), The EEG of Mental Activities,
pp. 42–49 (Karger, Basel 1988)

Quantitative EEG in the Diagnosis and Follow-Up of Alzheimer's Disease

Hilkka Soininen[a], *Juhani V. Partanen*[b]

[a] Department of Neurology, [b] Department of Clinical Neurophysiology,
Kuopio University Central Hospital, Kuopio, Finland

The final diagnosis of Alzheimer's disease (AD) is based on typical neuropathological findings at autopsy. So far there is no reliable peripheral marker of AD which could be used as a tool for definite diagnosis while living. The diagnosis of AD rests upon clinical assessment and exclusion of other causes of dementia. Using careful clinical evaluation the accuracy of AD diagnosis is at best 80–90% [9, 17]. A major problem in dementia diagnosis is to differentiate early AD from depression expressed as cognitive impairment, and from normal aging. In this respect also neurophysiological methods such as EEG, quantitative EEG and evoked potentials, have been used [2]. In some cases the follow-up of the patient will confirm the diagnosis, and quantitative EEG may further support the diagnosis. In drug trials in AD, quantitative EEG can be used to detect minor changes in brain functions. It is non-invasive, provides a direct sample of brain activity in a numerical form and is not influenced by motivational factors and practice effect as is neuropsychological examination [7, 13].

Slight EEG alterations are common in normal elderly people after the age of 60 years. The main changes are slowing of the alpha rhythm, appearance of slow activity and a theta focus in left temporal region [1, 8, 10, 11, 15]. However, the changes in EEG associated with aging are quite modest. Duffy et al. [6] suggested that previously reported age-related EEG slowing may be related to the presence of disease in the population studied.

EEG changes associated with AD consist of more slowing of the dominant occipital rhythm and more accentuation of theta and delta activity than is found in normal old people, but focal slowing occurs rarely [15].

In a recent paper, Coben et al. [3] point out that in mild AD the significant differences are accentuation of theta and decrease of beta activity and average mean frequency compared to matched normals. In a longitudinal study [4] of mild AD delta and theta increased and beta, alpha and mean frequency decreased during the study period of 2.5 years. In that study the theta percentage power distinguished between all 4 stages of dementia (control, mild, moderate, severe) while other EEG measures discriminated only at certain stages. In mild AD theta, beta and mean frequency were already different from control values. In the moderate stage, these differences persisted, and alpha became different. Delta was not different until in the severe stage of AD.

We have studied changes of quantitative EEG in different stages of AD. We also report some preliminary EEG data of a longitudinal follow-up study of early AD.

Methods

Forty-two patients with a presumptive diagnosis of AD (mean age 73 years, SD $\pm$ 8) and with different degrees of mental deterioration were chosen for the study. The diagnosis was based on clinical criteria [5]. Other causes of dementia were excluded by laboratory tests and CT scan of the brain, and patients included had 4 or less in Hachinski ischaemic score [14].

The stage of mental deterioration was determined by a neuropsychological test battery. The total score ranged from 0, representing complete failure, to 102, representing full marks. The AD patients were divided into 4 groups according to their scores: mild (70–91), moderate (51–69), marked (20–50) and severe (0–19) [14]. As controls, we studied healthy volunteers: 11 old people, aged 73 $\pm$ 7 years, and 11 young people, aged 33 $\pm$ 7 years.

In the longitudinal study we are following 33 patients with probable AD [12] from the early stage of dementia. We are using clinical rating scales, neuropsychological examinations and neurophysiological measures. Preliminary EEG data of one year's follow-up of 24 patients are reported.

We analysed either 16 or 32 s of waking artefact-free occipital EEG with eyes closed from T_5-O_1 or T_6-O_2 derivation. The EEG was fed to a Tracor Northern 1710 multichannel analyser through a 12-bit a/d converter using 8 ms sampling interval. The total epoch analysed was 32 s. The EEG samples were transferred to a Tektronix 4052 computer for fast Fourier transformation in 4-second epochs. The spectra were averaged before the final analysis. The integration formula is that of Penttilä et al. [14].

To calculate the mean frequency we used the frequency band 1.5–20.0 Hz according to the formula of Penttilä et al. [14]. It is a sensitive variable in mild AD. However, in order to seek the corresponding value for alpha activity (main power peak in EEG) we also calculated the mean frequency of a narrower band, 4.2–13.9 Hz. This variable is sensitive enough to differ significantly when old and young healthy adults are compared.

The percentage power of EEG in different frequency bands (beta, alpha, theta, delta) were calculated, as well as the mean and peak frequencies. The statistical analysis was performed with either the Student t test or the Mann-Whitney U-test.

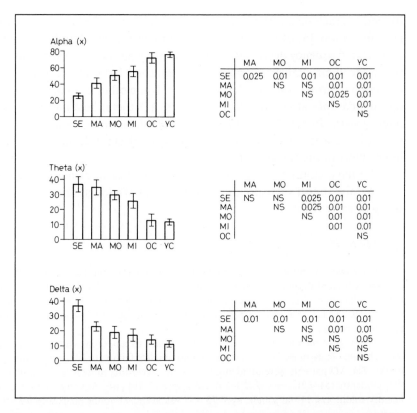

Fig. 1. The percentage power of the alpha, theta and delta bands (mean, SEM) of young (YC) and old controls (OC) and in mild (MI), moderate (MO), marked (MA) and severe (SE) AD. In the tables on the right there are the significances of differences (p <) between the different groups (Mann-Whitney U-test). Figures 1–3 are from Penttilä et al. [14] with permission.

Results

When the percentage powers of the alpha, theta and delta bands were compared, it was discovered that theta power increased in mild AD. The most marked increase in delta power did not occur until severe AD (compared with the old controls, fig. 1), and decrease of alpha power was significant in moderate but not in mild AD. The alpha/theta ratio decreased abruptly in mild AD, but the alpha/delta ratio decreased more linearly, and

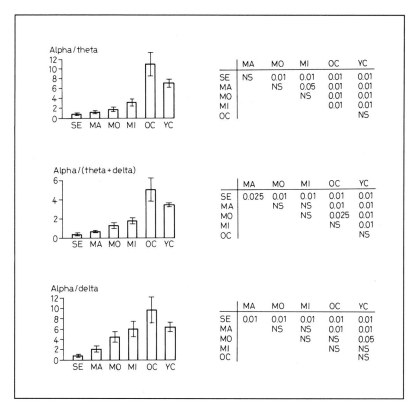

Fig. 2. The alpha/theta, the alpha/(theta + delta) and the alpha/delta ratios in controls and in different stages of AD. For abbreviations, see figure 1.

the difference was significant in marked and severe AD (compared with control values, fig. 2).

The occipital peak frequency was in the alpha band in mild and moderate AD and it was not significantly decreased in mild AD. The mean frequency was significantly decreased in mild AD (fig. 3). There was a significant correlation between the peak frequency and the neuropsychological test score ($r = 0.60$, $p < 0.001$). When old and young controls were compared the only significant difference was in the mean frequency (4.15–13.92 Hz; $p < 0.05$). The occipital peak frequency also tended to decrease.

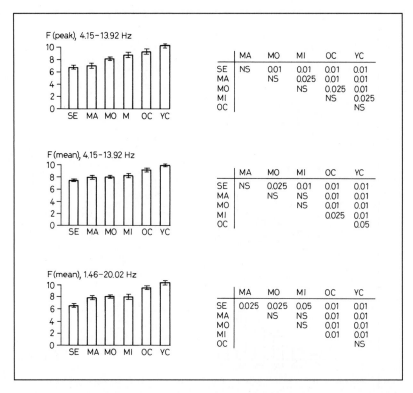

Fig. 3. The peak and the mean frequencies in controls and different stages of AD. For abbreviations, see figure 1.

The Longitudinal Study

When the EEG was recorded at baseline and after one year in 24 AD patients the following significant differences were found. The percentage power of alpha, the mean frequency in the range 1.5–20 Hz and the mean frequency in the range of alpha + theta decreased. The percentage of delta increased ($p < 0.01$). Beta + alpha/theta + delta ratio and the peak frequency decreased nearly significantly ($p < 0.05$). The percentage power of beta also tended to decrease, but not significantly. The percentage power of theta did not change.

When the EEG of individual patients were evaluated, it was evident that the EEG of 12 patients deteriorated markedly (fig. 4). There were 12

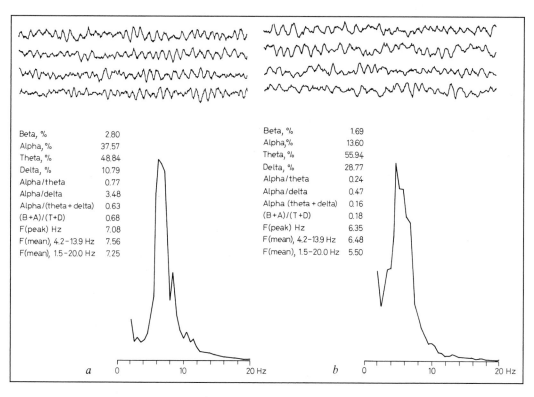

Beta, %	2.80
Alpha, %	37.57
Theta, %	48.84
Delta, %	10.79
Alpha/theta	0.77
Alpha/delta	3.48
Alpha/(theta + delta)	0.63
(B+A)/(T+D)	0.68
F(peak) Hz	7.08
F(mean), 4.2–13.9 Hz	7.56
F(mean), 1.5–20.0 Hz	7.25

Beta, %	1.69
Alpha, %	13.60
Theta, %	55.94
Delta, %	28.77
Alpha/theta	0.24
Alpha/delta	0.47
Alpha (theta + delta)	0.16
(B+A)/(T+D)	0.18
F(peak) Hz	6.35
F(mean), 4.2–13.9 Hz	6.48
F(mean), 1.5–20.0 Hz	5.50

Fig. 4. An epoch of occipital EEG and the power spectrum of the same EEG epoch of a patient with mild AD at baseline *(a)* and at one year *(b)*. Note deterioration of the values.

patients with a quite normal EEG at baseline and with minor or no changes between baseline and one-year recordings. Four of the patients with unchanged EEG had moderate dementia and 8 had mild dementia.

Discussion

When EEG changes in AD are discussed there are at least two factors to be considered: stage of dementia and the EEG measure studied. According to our findings variables which distinguish mild AD from controls are the percentage power of the theta band, the alpha/theta ratio and the mean frequency in the range 1.5–20.0 Hz. The percentage power of the alpha band, the occipital peak frequency and the alpha/delta ratio decreased linearly in different stages of AD. Distinct slowing of the occipital peak frequency and distinct accentuation of the percentage power of the delta band occurred in advanced AD. It is evident that slowing of the dominant occipital rhythm and accentuation of diffuse irregular slow waves describe rather advanced but not mild AD.

Our results agree with data of Coben et al. [3]. In the longitudinal study already at one year follow-up significant EEG changes appeared. Similar results were reported by Coben et al. [4]. An interesting finding is that there were several cases with normal EEG and no EEG deterioration during one year follow-up. There may be many explanations for this, i.e. variation in the natural course of the disease and also the limited accuracy of the clinical diagnosis. A patient with normal EEG and considerable dementia may prove to have Pick's disease at autopsy. Detailed analysis of clinical data of this study is in progress.

The value of the EEG in the differential diagnosis of dementia due to different causes is limited because the EEG reflects functional not structural changes in the brain [7]. Many disorders of the brain may produce similar EEG alterations. Thus reliable differential diagnosis cannot be made by using the EEG alone. However, the EEG can be used as a screening method to support differentiation between normal aging and dementia [16] and between dementia and depression. Quantitative EEG may be useful in follow-up of dementia patients and also in drug trials.

References

1 Busse, W.W.; Barnes, R.H.; Friedman, E.L.; Kelty, E.J.: Psychological functioning of aged individuals with normal and abnormal electroencephalograms. I. A study of nonhospitalised community volunteers. J. nerv. ment. Dis. *124:* 135–141 (1956).
2 Celesia, G.G.: EEG and event-related potentials in aging and dementia. J. clin. Neurophysiol. *3:* 99–111 (1986).
3 Coben, L.A.; Danziger, W.L.; Berg, L.: Frequency analysis of the resting awake EEG in mild senile dementia of Alzheimer type. Electroenceph. clin. Neurophysiol. *55:* 372–380 (1983).
4 Coben, L.A.; Danzinger, W.L.; Storandt, M.: A longitudinal EEG study of mild senile dementia of Alzheimer type: changes at 1 year and at 2.5 years. Electroenceph. clin. Neurophysiol. *61:* 101–112 (1985).
5 DSM III, American Psychiatric Association: Diagnostic and statistical manual of mental disorders; 3rd ed. (APA, Washington 1980).

6   Duffy, F.H.; Albert, M.S.; McAnulty, G.; Garvey, A.J.: Age-related differences in brain electrical activity of healthy subjects. Ann. Neurol. *16:* 430–438 (1984).
7   Fenton, G.W.: Electrophysiology of Alzheimer's disease. Br. med. Bull. *42:* 29–33 (1986).
8   Giaquinto, S.; Nolfe, G.: The EEG in the normal elderly: a contribution to the interpretation of aging and dementia. Electroenceph. clin. Neurophysiol. *63:* 540–546 (1986).
9   Katzman, R.: Alzheimer's disease. New Engl. J. Med. *314:* 964–973 (1986).
10 Levy, R.: The neurophysiology of dementia. Br. J. Psychiat. *9:* 119–123 (1975).
11 Matejcek, M.; Devos, J.E.: Selected methods of quantitative EEG analysis and their applications in phychotropic drug research; in Kellaway, Petersen, Quantitative analysic studies in epilepsy pp. 183–204 (Raven Press, New York 1976).
12 McKhann, G.; Drachman, D.; Folstein, M.; Katzman, R.; Price, D.; Stadlan, E.: Clinical diagnosis of Alzheimer's disease: report of the NINCDS-ADRDA Work Group under the auspices of Department of Health and Human Services Task Force on Alzheimer's disease. Neurology, Cleveland *34:* 939–944 (1984).
13 Partanen, V.J.; Soininen, H.; Riekkinen, P.J.: Does an ACTH derivative (Org 2766) prevent deterioration of EEG in Alzheimer's disease? Electroenceph. clin. Neurophysiol. *63:* 547–551 (1986).
14 Penttilä, M.; Partanen, V.J.; Soininen, H.; Riekkinen, P.J.: Quantitative analysis of occipital EEG in different stages of Alzheimer's disease. Electroenceph. clin. Neurophysiol. *60:* 1–6 (1985).
15 Soininen, H.; Partanen, V.J.; Helkala, E.-L.; Riekkinen, P.J.: EEG findings in senile dementia and normal aging. Acta neurol. scand. *65:* 59–70 (1982).
16 Soininen, H.; Partanen, V.J.; Puranen, M.; Riekkinen, P.J.: EEG and computed tomography in the investigation of patients with senile dementia. J. Neurol. Neurosurg. Psychiat. *45:* 711–714 (1982).
17 Sulkava, R.; Haltia, M.; Paetau, A.; Wikström, J.; Palo, J.: Accuracy of clinical diagnosis in primary degenerative dementia: correlation with neuropathological findings. J. Neurol. Neurosurg. Psychiat. *46:* 9–13 (1983).

H. Soininen, MD, Department of Neurology, Kuopio University Central Hospital, SF-70210 Kuopio (Finland)

Giannitrapani, Murri (eds.), The EEG of Mental Activities,
pp. 50–65 (Karger, Basel 1988)

The Electroencephalogram in the Elderly: Discrimination from Demented Patients and Correlation with CT Scan and Neuropsychological Data

A Review

Salvatore Giaquinto[a], *Giuseppe Nolfe*[b, 1]

[a] Ospedale San Giovanni Battista, SMOM, Roma;
[b] Istituto di Cibernetica CNR, Arco Felice, Italy

Electrical brain activity was discovered by Berger in 1929 but not until the 1950s did the first systematic studies of the aged [23] appear. A difference in the frequency of alpha rhythm in the aged was noted, 10.32 Hz in the control group and 9.39 Hz in subjects with an average age of 75 years. Among the tracings of the aged, 24% had anomalies of various types, but in other patients with signs of deterioration the value rose to 54%. A new study [31] stated that the background activity of the EEG in the elderly showed characteristics that would be abnormal if found in a young population. In a successive study [24], the alpha frequency of a healthy aged group had an average value of 9.16 Hz, while that of deteriorated subjects was around 8 Hz. Correlation with cerebral blood flow and brain metabolism was found only in the latter subjects, indicating that age is not responsible for EEG alterations. In the same study the fast beta activity was described as a characteristic of the aging process, with a decrease after the age period of 80s.

According to a study on demographic characteristics influencing the EEG of the elderly, the beta had a higher incidence in lower income classes, especially in women [39]. Furthermore, women had a more accelerated alpha frequency compared to men. Rapid activity was found in the tracings of all 10 subjects, from 100 years old and up. Discounting subjects

---

[1] Thanks are due to Sergio Piscitelli and Ciro Pierro for the computer analysis.

with generalized arteriosclerosis, an alpha rhythm with a frequency of 8.62 Hz was found. A 105-year-old subject showed a frequency of 9 Hz. The authors believe that no more noteworthy variations of EEG signals exist in the normal beyond 80 years [12].

Automatic analysis of the EEG permitted us to verify results already given here, and to deduct new information [8]. This type of analysis brings us from the time domain to the frequency domain: observations are not compiled from multiple pages, but on a cartesian diagram having the power on the ordinates and the frequency on the abscissae. Using the algorithm fast Fourier transform (FFT) in this analysis, the signal is divided into the frequencies of which it is formed. The first study of this type done with the aged showed a slight increase in relative power of the slow delta and theta bands, a slight decrease of the alpha and an increase of the faster activity, beta-2, that spans from 30 to 40 Hz [30]. The presence of these rhythms in the aged was considered positive by the author, as evidenced by the correlation with good mental capacity. A drop in the beta in the demented confirmed these data [3, 9].

Spectral variations were confirmed and a factor analysis was carried out on 619 normal subjects of different ages from 20 to 95 years, given a reciprocal dependency of EEG parameters and the presence of substructures not connected with aging [20]. Three factors accounted for 80% of the total variance; one was age-dependent. The age variable had the major role, immediately followed by alpha deceleration which represents the most characteristic sign of the senile EEG. Alpha rhythm shows a frequency slightly below 9 Hz, thus indicating a loss of about 1 Hz from youth to old age.

A lesser response to hyperventilation and to intermittent light stimulation was noticed along with the slowing of the alpha rhythm [13]. Reduced sensitivity to hyperventilation was not confirmed by Soininen et al. [32] who found a positive response in 66% of the cases. Probably, the different results to hyperventilation in the elderly depend on a different ventilation capacity instead of a different brain reactivity. For example, a recent study [4] showed positive response to hyperventilation in the aged only in 26% of the cases. Alpha rhythm reactivity decreased with age because its ratio in open and closed eyes conditions dropped linearly with age. The correlation coefficient is 0.434 significant at $p < 0.001$, 2-tailed.

The concept of alpha deceleration has been offset by recent observations, a condition similar to the doubts about some cognitive declines in the field of memory and problem solving. Studies conducted on the healthy aged contradict the concept of a marked slowing of EEG frequencies in the aging. In one of these studies [17], a high alpha frequency was found for the aged, i.e. 9.8 Hz. A frequency of 9.03 Hz was found by others with no difference due to sex [32]. Anomalies are present in a third of the subjects belonging to the aged group, but in Alzheimer's dementia the percentage rose to 94. Even the mildest case differentiated from the controls. Only 11% of the normal subjects showed asymmetries.

The study by Duffy et al. [4] denied the concept of a general slowing of EEG rhythms, perhaps because of accurate selection of the subjects. The alpha frequency showed no correlation with age; its amplitude, as well, had scarce correlation, while slow activity seemed to have a negative correlation. These authors also found an increase in fast rhythms but unfortunately did not specify the incidence in the two sexes.

An interesting study carried out on a middle-aged population, between 40 and 60 with an average age of 49 years, again diminished the significance of the percentages of abnormalities found in the aged [11]. These authors found a normal EEG tracing only in 39 of 170 healthy subjects (22.9%). The alpha frequency was 9.9 Hz, with extreme values of 8.6 and 11.2 Hz; 10% had an accentuated theta activity, 12% marked paroxysms and 34% slow temporal activity. Anomalies in the normal aged were seen in temporal derivations, especially on the left side. The data reveal a continuum among youth, middle-aged and aged with a stable EEG tracing, even at 100 years.

In one of our studies [9] comparing a sample group of aged with another of normal subjects between 40 and 60, no significant differences resulted. This observation indicates that the declining function has such a small derivative, it does not even appear when 2 age-adjacent cohorts are compared. We hold, along with others [18, 24, 33], that the general or, as happens more often, the focal alterations are not caused by age but by slight pathological alterations that can occur at any age, though they are more frequently found in older people. To the contrary, there is no valid way to explain the prevalence of focal slow activity in the left temporal area [2]. Other observations describe asymmetries with prevalence to the right, although emphasizing a good persistency of the electrical activity in the aged brain [4]. Relaxing techniques such as biofeedback can increase alpha rhythm percentage in the elderly, not its frequency. However, biofeedback alone does not produce more alpha than the usual instructions for a calm and image-maker mental state [2].

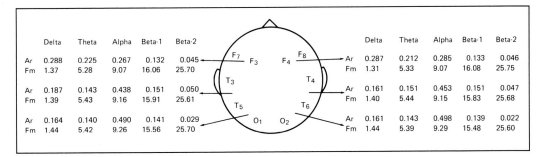

Fig. 1. Mean values of relative activity and weighted frequency for each of the five spectral bands on the leads F_3–F_7, T_3–T_5, T_5–O_1 and F_4–F_8, T_4–T_6, T_6–O_2.

Our work group has tried to verify through spectral analysis the distribution of EEG frequencies on the scalp and the differences from EEG katterns recorded in cases of Alzheimer's dementia [9]. In general, the literature mainly considers the occipital activity which is highest in alpha rhythm. At the same time, a question arises as to whether regional differentiation has been kept, since temporal, parietal and frontal areas are known anatomically to be more affected than the occipital area. In a group of healthy subjects (n = 47, mean age 71 years), who lacked any therapy as well as hypnotics, the alpha frequency shows a topographical localization with simultaneous intrahemispherical symmetry, as confirmed in other studies [38]. Pairing left and right, we found the following values: 9.07 and 9.07 in the frontal areas, 9.16 and 9.15 in the temporal areas, and 9.26 and 9.29 in the occipital areas. The values of the 5 bands of the spectrum are listed in figure 1. As an interesting consequence, we deduct the preservation of a functional structure in the normal aging, where the regional differences already observed in the adult for the various areas are respected. Alpha rhythm is shown with a frequency of 9 Hz or more, also in frontal areas, though they are the poorest.

Concerning sex differences, from our research came the prevalence in men of the delta rhythm, the slowest, and the prevalence in women of the beta rhythm, the fastest (fig. 2). As mentioned previously, this difference was described years ago through visual EEG inspection. It appears that men are more affected than women by the aging process, at least from the electrophysiological point of view, because slow frequencies have a negative correlation with cognitive tasks, while fast frequencies bear the opposite relationship, as will be reported later.

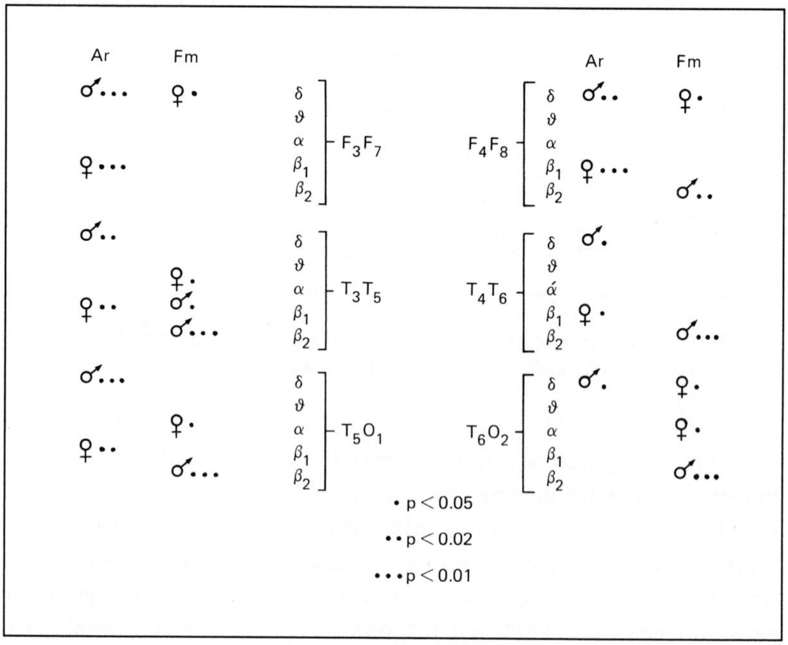

Fig. 2. The sex-prevalence is listed for two spectral parameters (relative activity, Ar, and mean frequency, Fm) on each of the five bands. The dots indicate the significance levels. Same channels as in figure 1. For example, in the channel F_3–F_7 it is evident that a strong prevalence of delta relative activity exists in men, while a strong prevalence of beta activity exists in women. Women in that channel also have a faster delta frequency. Beta activity is prevalent in women on 5 channels out of 6. Delta activity is prevalent in men on 6 channels out of 6. Men have a lesser amount of beta activity, but a higher frequency on that band.

In a comparison between the normal aged and demented [37] anomalies were found in 52 and 82% of the cases, respectively. This difference is very sharp, although the indicated 52% of abnormalities appears higher than literature usually reports. However, for the authors who include 50-year-old subjects in their research, anomalies appear to be slight (37.7%) and moderate (16.3%). Comparison of aged versus demented greatly improves with EEG spectral analysis. The parameters of delta and theta relative activities, which increase in dementia, and those of alpha and beta, which decrease, are generally considered significant [9, 28, 38]. Figures 3 and 4 display significant differences among 3 groups of subjects, middle-

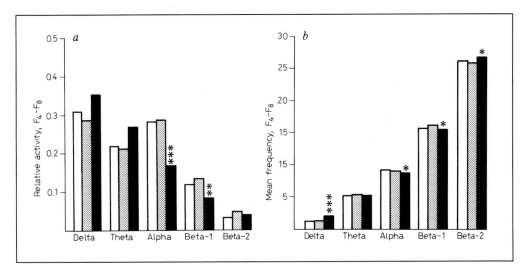

Fig. 3. Channel F_4–F_8, five frequency bands. On the y-axis the relative activity (a) and the mean frequency (b) are shown for three cohorts: middle-aged (empty column), normal elderly (horizontal bars) and demented subjects (vertical lines). * $p < 0.05$; ** $p < 0.02$; *** $p < 0.01$. From Giaquinto and Nolfe [9].

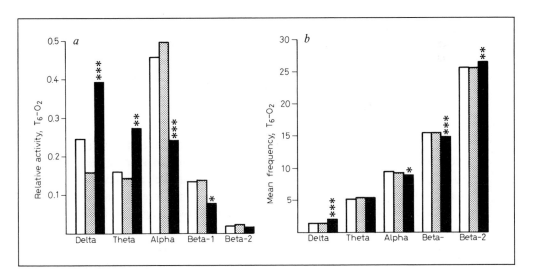

Fig. 4. Channel T_6–O_2. Same indications as in figure 3. Demented patients display increase of delta and theta relative activity with decrease of alpha and beta activity. Shifts in frequency are also significant. From Giaquinto and Nolfe [9].

Table I. Values of the correlation coefficient between age and mean weighted frequency. Class of age: 60–80 years. N = 32 alpha-dominant subjects

Derivation	Delta	Theta	Alpha	Beta-1	Beta-2
F_3–F_7 (left frontal)	−0.198	0.492**	−0.376*	−0.04	−0.391*
F_4–F_8 (right frontal)	0.115	0.416*	−0.385*	0.295	−0.273
T_3–T_5 (left middle temporal)	−0.022	0.325	−0.407*	−0.02	−0.034
T_4–T_6 (right middle temporal)	0.08	0.221	−0.389*	−0.21	−0.03
T_5–O_1 (left temporo-occipital)	−0.130	0.353*	−0.303	−0.23	0.181
T_6–O_2 (right temporo-occipital)	0.021	0.447*	−0.351	−0.31	0.131

* $p < 0.05$; ** $p < 0.01$.

Table II. Values of the correlation coefficient between age and relative activity. Class of age: 60–80 years. N = 32 alpha-dominant subjects

Derivation	Delta	Theta	Alpha	Beta-1	Beta-2
F_3–F_7 (left frontal)	0.244	0.08	−0.146	−0.203	−0.405*
F_4–F_8 (right frontal)	−0.1	0.202	−0.045	−0.103	−0.01
T_3–T_5 (left middle temporal)	0.047	0.436*	−0.091	−0.272	−0.138
T_4–T_6 (right middle temporal)	0.097	0.466**	−0.238	−0.243	−0.013
T_5–O_1 (left temporo-occipital)	0.185	0.464**	−0.244	−0.140	−0.153
T_6–O_2 (right temporo-occipital)	0.229	0.444*	−0.177	−0.258	−0.241

* $p < 0.05$; ** $p < 0.01$.

aged, aged and mildly demented. Differences among the groups are very clear in the frontal and temporal areas. The reduction of average frequency of the total spectrum is also discriminating [38], as well as some parameters of event-related potentials that will not be considered in this article.

Calculation of the correlation coefficient between age and EEG spectral parameters gave the values of tables I and II. Alpha frequency is negatively correlated with age, while theta frequency is correlated positively. Concerning relative activity, a significant correlation was found for the theta band only, especially in temporal areas.

In the normal elderly there are cases of EEG alterations, which are generally focal. We must consider that: (1) percentage incidence in a normal aged group is significantly lower than the group of aged subjects with neurological problems; (2) these anomalies are also noticed in much younger normal subjects, where ordinarily the diagnosis of deterioration would be very unlikely. Data in the latter subjects show quite frequent shifts from canonic values. The early conclusions [24] were confirmed in a study conducted on subjects under 64 years of age, where abnormal tracings were not dependent on the 'age' variable [22]. There are EEG data that appear useful in differentiating the natural aging process and that are caused by dementia [3, 25]. In the latter condition, the alpha rhythm only in the early phase reduces and flattens out, to be replaced by slow diffuse rhythms with eventual paroxysms. The EEG changes appear to be more helpful in suspecting or diagnosing cases of Alzheimer's dementia than CT-scan modifications and they are also early signs [1]. In doubtful cases it is advisable to record a new tracing after 3 months and to match computerized values. It has been found that the test-retest procedure indicates a good reliability of the alpha frequency, at least in children [5]. In many cases there can be a false-negative EEG [19], while, according to other authors [10], the tracing is always pathological in Alzheimer's dementia, in contrast to that of Pick's dementia. Measures involving both resting EEG and evoked response conditions discriminated with 82% accuracy cognitively impaired elderly subjects from a control group matched for sex, race, age and education [15]. A recent study [28] supports the thesis of early EEG alterations in cases of mild Alzheimer's dementia. They mainly affect the percentage power of the theta band, the ratio of powers in the alpha and theta bands and the mean frequency (range 1.46–20.02 Hz). There appears to be no close relationship between the seriousness of the disease and the extent of the EEG damage [10], but other authors argue that the more abnormal the tracing, the more deteriorated the cognitive functions [14].

The correlation of the CT-scan data with the EEG data is not proved. No correlation resulted between the presence and the seriousness of EEG abnormalities and the degree of brain atrophy, as observed by evaluation of the distance between the most lateral points of the frontal horns and of the width of the third ventricle [34], or else automatically with three relationships between parenchima and liquoral spaces on three sections [7]. In this study, although the EEG correlates neither with the CT-scan data nor with age, it can be correlated with the mental decline. On the contrary, the ventricular volume correlates with age instead of decline. Further results have been reported on this line: the EEG delta frequency does not correlate with the ventricular dilatation but does with the cognitive impairment [1,

29]. From these observations one can see the EEG contribution to the study of the brain aging and decline as being more essential with respect to that of the CT scan. Such a conclusion is in fact supported by another study that includes CT scan, EEG and neuropsychological testing on 78 subjects with suspected deterioration, without overt neurological focal signs or other evident organic brain illness [16]. The main result shows in fact that the most reliable parameter is the EEG slowing.

We can therefore conclude that the normal EEG tracing in the elderly maintains the same general characteristics as in the young controls. Spectral analysis with a frequency resolution of 0.25 Hz shows that the frequency and the power of alpha rhythm on the brain cortex of the aged maintain a somatotopic distribution, with higher values on the occipital areas. Left and right comparison does not show significant side difference, at least on the basis of the power spectrum. There is a good agreement among the authors on the value of the alpha frequency in the elderly (table III), both with visual inspection and automatic analysis. The slowing down in the aged is certainly restricted to a maximum of 1 Hz.

The last topic of this article deals with the intriguing problem of the correlations between EEG and mental activities. This topic is discussed in this book by other colleagues and therefore we are going to briefly report some data in the framework of the aging brain.

The research in this field had no particular advances, mainly for the relative usefulness of the WAIS scale in the elderly, which was not considered a specially designed testing by Wechsler himself. However, in a group of 32 healthy subjects who also underwent EEG recording, no significant changes were seen on the WAIS in a study made 3.5 years after the initial examination, thus indicating a good mental stability [40]. A timing mechanism was also hypothesized to explain the parallel slowing down of the alpha rhythm and of the cognitive performances [35, 36], as if the alpha band were a sort of timer. A crude scepticism against any correlation between EEG was then expressed, especially concerning the alpha rhythm and psychological functions [6].

The concept that the resting EEG can be considered as a monitor of the integrity of the underlying cortex is the basis for the endeavor of other authors to find significant correlations with cognitive functioning in the elderly. The possibility of quantitative data sets brought about by computerized EEG added more interest to the problem. A correlation matrix between EEG and some psychological variables shows very low but nevertheless significant coefficients, indicating that vigilance has a connection

Table III. Alpha mean frequency in the elderly (Hz)

Mundy-Castle et al.	9.39
Obrist et al.	9.16
Otomo	9.47
Wang and Busse	9.08 (M)
	9.44 (F)
Harner	9.40
Hubbard et al.	9.56*
Hughes and Cayaffa	9.00**
Soininen et al.	9.03
Katz and Horowitz	9.80
Torres et al.	9.70
Visser et al.	9.60
Giaquinto and Nolfe	9.07 (frontal)
	9.15 (temporal)
	9.29 (occipital)

* Data from centenarians.
** Approximated values.

from one side with EEG frequencies and on the other side with perceptual and mental activities [26]. In a population of active and bright aged women from parietal leads the so-called sigma band (13.2–14.8 Hz) is found to be related to superior cognitive functions in a study, where mainly the WAIS score is used [27]. In the same study, the other consistent correlations were those between bilateral theta activity and Bender Gestalt copying; between Wechsler Memory Scale mental control and bilateral slow alpha activity.

In another study, EEG was recorded under different mental activation, such as listening to a tale or music, recalling or recognizing abstract figures, reading or recalling paired associates [4]. EEG features were obtained that can be described in terms of (1) cortical region; (2) behavioral state; (3) frequency band; (4) raw or normalized data. All temporal lobe features derived from EEG slow activity are positively correlated with measures of memory, where features derived from fast activity were negatively correlated. The association of higher memory scores with larger amounts of delta and theta and smaller amount of beta is apparently surprising. Probably, the association is not explained by the frequencies but rather by the functional state, because the EEG was simultaneously recorded. In a retrospective study significant correlation coefficients were found for as many as 10 of the 19 SCAG items and two of the five SCAG factors with at least one of the four EEG variables [21]. In this study deterioration in most of the SCAG items and factors correlating with the resting EEG shows an increase in the slow activity. For example, significant ($p < 0.05$) Spearman rank correlation coefficients are found; the correlation in this case is always positive. As it is known, the absence of a sign or a symptom is scored 1 at the SCAG scale, while the worst condition is scored 7.

In order to bring a contribution to the problem of the significance of a correlation study we recorded the EEG in 47 elderly people. The sample consisted of 32 men and 15 women without any history of neurological diseases, who were untreated by drugs and lived at their home, with regular activities and social relations. The mean age of the cohort was 71.08 with a standard deviation of 5.86. The range was 60–80 years. All were right-handed and had normal, or corrected, visual acuity. They took part in the investigation on invitation. EEG was taken in the morning after breakfast in a sound-attenuated room. Ag/AgCl cup electrodes were fixed according to the 10–20 system. The signals were amplified and filtered through a band from 0.2 to 40 Hz. Six derivations were stored on magnetic tape for computerized analysis. They were: F_3-F_7, T_3-T_5, T_5-O_1; F_4-F_8, T_4-T_6, T_6-O_2. A seventh channel on the tape was allotted for a digital code. One hundred and twenty cumulative seconds of artifact-free tracings were selected and fed to an A/D converter.

Following a sampling rate of 128/s, the FFT was used for the calculation of the spectral density functions. Spectral characteristics were the following: resolution 0.25 Hz, normalized standard error 0.18. For each band two spectral descriptors were applied: relative activity (Ar); mean weighted frequency (Fm). The bands were classified as delta (0.25–3.75 Hz), theta (4–7.75 Hz), alpha (8–12.25), beta-1 (12.50–20 Hz) and finally beta-2 (20.25–32 Hz).

Neuropsychological testing was performed the next day. Tachistoscopy (TS) and reaction times were measured by utilizing a specially built microprocessing apparatus. Subjects sat in a comfortable position in front of a display which subtended a visual angle of 8°. The following performances were measured: (1) TS for colors: yellow, blue, red. (2) TS for sharp patterns, with neat edges. (3) TS for shaded patterns, having less defined contrast from the background. (4) TS for 5-letter words of high frequency. (5) TS for random 5-digit numbers. (6) Simple reaction time to a red flash. (7) Choice reaction time, based on visual discrimination

Table IV. Paced and nonpaced neuropsychological testing

Tachistoscopy for a	young controls	21	(100)
meaningful 5-letter word	elderly normal subjects	313***	(100)
	demented patients	3,257***	(43)
Tachistoscopy for a	young controls	42	(100)
5-digit number	elderly normal subjects	1,083***	(100)
	demented patients	6,050***	(21)
Pattern recognition	young controls	28	(100)
(shaded pattern)	elderly normal subjects	639***	(100)
	demented patients	5,782***	(64)
Choice reaction time	young controls	327	(100)
	elderly normal subjects	482***	(100)
	demented patients	987***	(64)
Free recall	young controls	13.54	
(Rey verbal test, trial 5)	elderly normal subjects	10.37***	
	demented patients	2.43***	
Delayed recall	young controls	12.58	
	elderly normal subjects	8.67***	
	demented patients	0.64***	
Block tapping test	young controls	6.55	
	elderly normal subjects	4.85***	
	demented patients	1.13***	

Paced tasks have mean values expressed in milliseconds. The percentage of capable subjects is given in parentheses.
*** $p < 0.001$.
Paired comparison: controls vs elderly subjects, elderly vs demented patients.

between 2 colors. (8) Rey test for verbal memory. (9) Block tapping test, for spatial memory. The visual stimuli on the monitor had a minimum frame time of 18 ms with steps of 18 ms up to a maximum of 17.9 s. Subjects were stimulated binocularly. Precautions were taken to avoid image persistence on the phosphor of the screen. The visual angles subtended by colors and patterns were respectively 8 and 6°, those subtended by letters and numbers were respectively 1° 20' in the vertical and 58' in the horizontal axis. The lighting was 0.2 lux, full-moon type, clearly visible but not dazzling, with 100% of contrast. For measuring reaction times the subject had to press his right hand on a conveniently situated knob.

Table V. Correlations: EEG – neuropsychological tests

6 channels	F_3–F_7, T_3–T_5, T_5–O_1; F_4–F_8, T_4–T_6, T_6–O_1
5 spectral bands	delta, theta, alpha, beta-1, beta-2
2 spectral parameters	mean frequency, relative power
7 tests	words and numbers tachistoscopy
	pattern recognition
	choice reaction time
	free recall
	block tapping
	delayed recall

Total number of possible correlation coefficients: $6 \times 5 \times 2 \times 7 = 420$. Significant correlation coefficients: 33 at 0.05 level of significance. Correlation coefficients due to change: 16.

Data obtained from this neuropsychological testing are shown in table IV. The performance of the elderly subjects is maintained in some tests compared to younger controls, such as the tachistoscopy for colors and sharp pattern (not shown here), whereas it is quantitatively different in experiments involving paced tasks or excessive memory load.

Our observations on both EEG and neuropsychological data collected from the same subjects suggest that true correlations do exist and that the findings are not due to mere chance. Results are shown in table V.

The problem of the correlation between cortical electrical activity and mental operations is intriguing but tricky. Since the statistical analysis consists of numerous correlations, a certain number of them would appear to be significant by chance alone. It is the consistency of the patterns, their formal significance, their interpretation on the basis of previous and parallel findings which can give the correlation coefficients, as a whole, reliability and scientific dignity.

References

1   Angeleri, F.; Provinciali, L.; Signorino, M.; Piana, C.; Salvolini, U.: Ageing mind, depression and dementia: a neuropsychological, electrophysiological and CT approach to the clinical diagnosis; in Cecchini, Nappi, Arrigo, Cerebral pathology in old age, pp. 91–102 (Emiras, Pavia 1983).

2   Busse, E.W.: Electroencephalography; in Reisberg, Alzheimer's disease: The standard reference, pp. 231–237 (Free Press, New York 1983).
3   Coben, L.A.; Danzinger, W.L.; Berg, L.: Frequency analysis of the resting awake
    EEG in mild senile dementia of Alzheimer type. Electroenceph. clin. Neurophysiol.
    55: 372–380 (1983).
4   Duffy, F.H.; Albert, M.S.; McAnulty, G.; Garvey, A.J.: Age-related differences in
    brain electrical activity of healthy subjects. Ann. Neurol. 16: 430–438 (1984).
5   Gasser, T.; Bacher, P.; Steinberg, H.: Test-retest reliability of spectral parameters of
    the EEG. Electroenceph. clin. Neurophysiol. 60: 312–319 (1985).
6   Gastaut, H.: Vom Berger-Rhythmus zum Alpha-Kult und zur Alpha-Kultur. EEG-
    EMG 5: 189–199 (1974).
7   Gastaut, J.L.; Farnarier, G.; Michel, B.; Serbanescu, T.; Barrat, E.; Sambuc, R.:
    Etude correlative des données EEG et scanographiques au cours du vieillissement
    cérébral normal et pathologique. Rev. EEG Neurophysiol. 10: 228–235 (1980).
8   Giaquinto, S.: Computerized EEG in the study of cerebral alteration and brain
    pathology in the aged; in Barbagallo-Sangiorgi, Exton-Smith, The aging brain, pp.
    229–239 (Plenum Press, New York 1980).
9   Giaquinto, S.; Nolfe, G.: The EEG in the normal elderly: a contribution to the
    interpretation of aging and dementia. Electroenceph. clin. Neurophysiol. 63: 540–
    546 (1986).
10 Gordon, E.B.; Sim, M.: The EEG in presenile dementia. J. Neurol. Neurosurg. Psychiat. 30: 285–291 (1967).
11 Guggenheim, P.; Karbowski, K.: EEG-Befunde bei 40–60jährigen gesunden Probanden. Z. Gerontol. 12: 365–375 (1979).
12 Hubbard, O.; Sunde, D.; Goldensohn, E.S.: The EEG in centenarians. Electroenceph. clin. Neurophysiol. 40: 407–417 (1976).
13 Hughes, J.R.; Cayaffa, J.J.: The EEG in patients at different ages without organic
    cerebral disease. Electroenceph. clin. Neurophysiol. 42: 776–784 (1977).
14 Johannesson, G.; Hagberg, B.; Gustafson, L.; Ingvar, D.H.: EEG and cognitive
    impairment in presenile dementia. Acta neurol. scand. 59: 225–240 (1979).
15 John, E.R.; Karmel, B.Z.; Corning, W.C.; Easton, P.; Brown, D.; Ahn, H.; John, M.;
    Harmony, T.; Prichep, L.; Toro, A.; Gerson, I.; Bartless, F.; Thatcher, R.; Kaye, H.;
    Valdes, P.; Schartz, E.E.: Neurometrics. Science 210: 1255–1258 (1977).
16 Kaszniak, A.W.; Garron, D.C.; Fox, J.H.; Bergen, D.; Huckman, M.: Cerebral atrophy, EEG slowing age, education and cognitive functioning in suspected dementia.
    Neurology 29: 1273–1279 (1979).
17 Katz, R.I.; Horowitz, G.R.: Electroencephalogram in the septuagenarians: studies in
    a normal geriatric population. J. Am. Geriat. Soc. 3: 273–275 (1982).
18 Kazis, A.; Karlovasitou, A.; Xafenias, D.: Temporal slow activities of the EEG in old
    age. Arch. Psychiat. NervKrankh. 231: 547–554 (1982).
19 Liston, E.H.: Clinical findings in presenile dementia. J. nerv. ment. Dis. 167: 337–
    342 (1979).
20 Matejcek, M.: Application de l'analyse spectrale pour l'étude de certaines relations
    entre l'activité EEG occipitale et l'âge. Rev. EEG Neurophysiol. 10: 122–130
    (1980).

21 Matejcek, M.; Blasowitsch, R.; Schweingruber, M.; Abt, K.: Some correlations in geriatric patients between EEG parameters and clinical status as evaluated using the observer-rated SCAG rating scale; in Mendlewicz, Pull, Janke, Kunkel, Neuropsychobiology, No. 15, pp. 49–56 (Karger, Basel 1986).

22 Matousek, M.; Volavka, J.; Roubicek, J.; Roth, Z.: EEG frequency analysis related to age in normal adults. Electroenceph. clin. Neurophysiol. 23: 162–167 (1967).

23 Mundy-Castle, A.; Hurst, L.A.; Beerstecher, D.; Prinsloo, T.: The electroencephalogram in the senile psychoses. Electroenceph. clin. Neurophysiol. 6: 245–252 (1954).

24 Obrist, W.D.; Sokoloff, L.; Lassen, N.A.; Lane, M.H.; Butler, R.N.; Feinberg, I.: Relation of EEG to cerebral blood flow and metabolism in old age. Electroenceph. clin. Neurophysiol. 15: 610–619 (1963).

25 Ono, K.; Mameda, G.; Shimada, D.; Yamashita, M.: EEG correlation with intelligence test performance in senescence: a new pattern discriminative approach. Int. J. Neurosci. 16: 47–52 (1982).

26 Ott, H.; McDonald, R.J.; Fichte, K.; Herrmann, W.M.: Interpretation of correlation between EEG-power-spectra and psychological performance variables within the concepts of subvigilance, attention and psychomotoric impulsion; in Herrmann, Electroencephalography in drug research, pp. 227–247 (Fischer, Stuttgart 1982).

27 Patterson, M.B.; Gluck, H.; Mack, J.L.: EEG activity in the 13–15 Hz band correlates with intelligence in healthy elderly women. Int. J. Neurosci. 20: 161–172 (1983).

28 Penttila, M.; Partanen, J.V.; Soininen, H.; Riekkinen, P.J.: Quantitative analysis of occipital EEG in different stages of Alzheimer's disease. Electroenceph. clin. Neurophysiol. 60: 1–6 (1985).

29 Roberts, M.A.; McGeorge, A.P.; Caird, F.I.: Electroencephalography and computerized tomography in vascular and non-vascular dementia in old age. J. Neurol. Neurosurg. Psychiat. 41: 903–906 (1978).

30 Roubicek, J.: The electroencephalogram in the middle-aged and the elderly. J. Am. Geriat. Soc. 25: 145–152 (1977).

31 Silverman, A.J.; Busse, E.W.; Barnes, R.H.: Studies in the process of aging: electroencephalographic findings in 400 elderly subjects. Electroenceph. clin. Neurophysiol. 7: 67–74 (1955).

32 Soininen, H.; Partanen, V.J.; Helkala, E.L.; Riekkinen, P.J.: EEG findings in senile dementia and normal aging. Acta neurol. scand. 65: 59–70 (1982).

33 Sokoloff, L.: Cerebral circulatory and metabolic changes associated with aging. Res. Publ. Ass. nerv. ment. Dis. 41: 237–254 (1966).

34 Stefoski, D.; Bergen, D.; Fox, J.; Morrell, F.; Huckman, M.; Ramsey, R.: Correlation between diffuse EEG abnormalities and cerebral atrophy in senile dementia. J. Neurol. Neurosurg. Psychiat. 39: 751–755 (1976).

35 Surwillo, W.W.: The relation to simple response time to brain wave frequency and the effect of age. Electroenceph. clin. Neurophysiol. 15: 105–114 (1963).

36 Surwillo, W.W.: The relation of decision time to brain wave frequency and old age. Electroenceph. clin. Neurophysiol. 16: 510–514 (1964).

37 Torres, F.; Faoro, A.; Loewenson, R.; Johnson, E.: The electroencephalogram of elderly subjects revisited. Electroenceph. clin. Neurophysiol. 56: 391–398 (1983).

38   Visser, S.L.; Van Tilburg, W.; Hooijer, C.; Jonker, C.; De Rijke, W.: Visual evoked
     potentials (VEPS) in senile dementia (Alzheimer type) and in nonorganic behav-
     ioural disorders in the elderly: comparison with EEG parameters. Electroenceph.
     clin. Neurophysiol. *60:* 115–121 (1985).
39   Wang, H.S.; Busse, E.W.: EEG of healthy old persons – a longitudinal study. I.
     Dominant background activity and occipital rhythm. J. Geront. *24:* 419–426
     (1969).
40   Wang, H.S.; Obrist, W.D.; Busse, E.W.: Neurophysiological correlates of the intel-
     lectual function; in Palmore, Normal aging II, pp. 115–126 (Duke University Press,
     Durham 1974).

Salvatore Giaquinto, MD, Ospedale San Giovanni Battista, SMOM,
I–00148 Roma (Italy)

Giannitrapani, Murri (eds.), The EEG of Mental Activities,
pp. 66–74 (Karger, Basel 1988)

EEG and Dementia in Hereditary Cerebral Haemorrhage with Amyloidosis

Gudjon Johannesson, Gunnar Gudmundsson

Department of Neurology, National Hospital, University of Iceland, Reykjavik, Iceland

Hereditary cerebral haemorrhage with amyloidosis (HCHWA) is an autosomal dominant disease affecting young adults. The disease is known only in Iceland where it formerly was confined to an area in the western part of the country [1, 11]. A similar condition affecting older age groups has been described in the Netherlands [23, 31]. In about 90% of the cases the onset of symptoms is between 15 and 50 years, but in a small percentage the condition apparently is compatible with reaching old age. The death rate from HCHWA is highest in the third decade. The age of death in 59 males and 63 females is shown in figure 1 [16]. The transmission of the disease in a family is shown in figure 2.

It has been shown that the amyloid fibril in HCHWA is related to the neuroendocrine microprotein cystatin C (gamma-trace) [5]. Further, it has been demonstrated that the CSF level of cystatin C in HCHWA is significantly reduced (<4 mg/l) [10], and the molecule differs from the normal type of cystatin C, possibly because of a point mutation [9]. About 80% of the patients have organic mental symptoms and in some cases dementia is the presenting symptom of the disease [12], but apparently practically all those who do not die from the first attacks become demented.

HCHWA is one of the cerebral amyloidoses in which the protein component has been isolated and characterized. The other two are Alzheimer's disease and the unconventional virus diseases ('slow virus diseases') of which Jacob-Creutzfeldt disease is one [24].

Most types of organic dementia are associated with EEG changes. This was first noted by Berger [2] in a patient who on autopsy proved to have

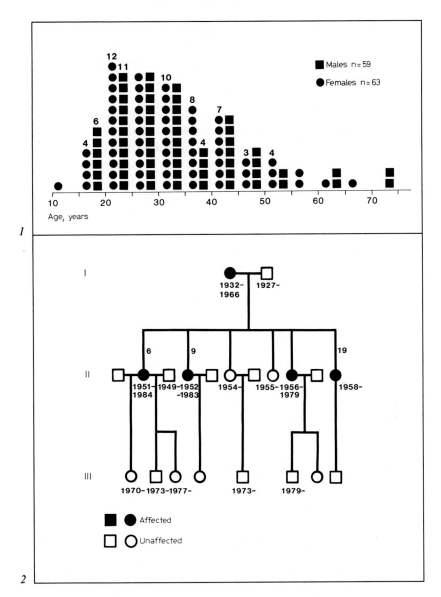

Fig. 1. One hundred and twenty-two patients with HCHWA. Sex distribution and age at death. From [16] with permission from Plenum Publishing Corporation.

Fig. 2. A family with HCHWA. Generations are marked with Roman numerals. Cases No. 6, 9 and 19 who are included in this material, are specially marked. Year of birth and year of death respectively are indicated below the individual symbols. The dominance of females in this family is accidental.

Alzheimer's disease. In Alzheimer's disease there is a successive slowing and loss of alpha activity, and in studies on histologically proven Alzheimer cases the proportion of abnormal EEG approaches 100% [6, 18, 20]. Similar, but less pronounced changes, have been reported in the EEG of patients with senile dementia [7].

Jacob-Creutzfeldt's disease, in advanced cases, often shows specific changes with bilateral rhythmic complexes [4, 8, 19]. It should be mentioned here that in the acquired immune deficiency syndrome (AIDS) which is a slow virus disease in which dementia is common and may be the first symptom, the EEG is often abnormal [3, 21, 26].

In the dementia of cerebrovascular disease (CVD, MID, multi-infarct dementia) the changes are more often localized and a number of such patients have normal EEG [13, 17, 18, 27]. In Pick's disease the EEG often is normal on conventional visual inspection [18, 30], even if automatic analysis may detect frontal abnormality [29]. In Huntington's chorea a low voltage EEG is often found [28].

Material and Methods

During the last 25 years EEG recordings have been done on a number of HCHWA patients although there has been no systematic EEG study. This is a report on the EEG of 22 patients belonging to families with known HCHWA. Figure 2 shows a family of which 3 members are included in this study (cases 6, 9, and 19 in fig. 3 and table I). Seventeen of the 22 subjects have died from cerebral haemorrhage. In 8 of these a measurement of the cystatin C level in the CSF had been done [10] and in all cases found to be abnormally low (table I). Those 5 who are still alive have unequivocal symptoms of a CNS affection and all of them have reduced cystatin C level in the CSF (table I). In most cases records taken after 1965 could be retrieved for direct evaluation. In a few cases, however, only the EEG report was available so that the classification was based on that. The classification in table II, however, is in all cases based on existing EEG records.

Most of the EEG recordings were done on a 16- or 8-channel Kaiser EEG equipment, a small number on an 8-channel Grass machine. The lower frequency limit was 0.3 and the higher 70 Hz. The electrode placement was according to the international 10–20 system [15] using a bipolar recording. When possible the patient was awake and at rest with closed eyes. Hyperventilation and photic stimulation were included when possible. The records were classified by means of conventional visual inspection and divided into 4 classes: E0 = normal; E1 = slightly abnormal; E2 = moderately abnormal; E3 = severely abnormal. The criteria for the classification were as follows: slightly abnormal records contained a small quantity of episodic or diffuse 4–7 Hz activity with an amplitude not exceeding 100 µV. Moderately abnormal EEG contained a greater quantity of 4–7 Hz activity and/or some diffuse delta activity. Severely abnormal EEGs were dominated by delta and theta activity. Often the abnormality was asymmetrical. On the other hand focal

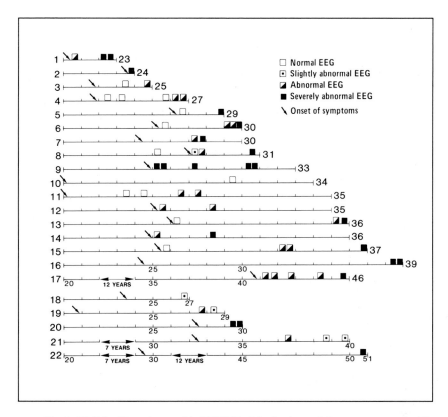

Fig. 3. EEG in 22 patients with HCHWA. The horizontal lines represent the life span after 20. In a few cases the time scale had to be modified because of an exceptionally long duration of disease in cases 17, 21 and 22. Onset of disease is indicated by an oblique arrow. Individual EEG records are represented by squares as explained in the picture. The figure after the end of each of the first 17 horizontal lines indicates age at death. The figure under the termination of each of the last 5 horizontal lines shows the approximate age in years in January 1987.

and paroxysmal features were rather uncommon. All records were classified by the same physician (G.J.).

Dementia and other mental symptoms were, in all cases, assessed by one of us (G.G.). In case 6 the absence of dementia was confirmed by psychological testing which showed an above average intelligence (IQ 118). The group was divided according to the degree of dementia into 4 classes: D0 = no mental deterioration; D1 = mild dementia, consisting of mild memory disturbances and/or mild dysphasia; D2 = moderate dementia, with moderate memory loss and general intellectual reduction; D3 = severe dementia with memory loss, disorientation, dysphasia and dyspraxia.

Results

Figure 3 summarizes some clinical and EEG findings in 22 patients with HCHWA of whom 17 have died from the disease. It can be seen that the duration of disease is very variable. In one of these cases the first

Table I. Some clinical findings in 22 patients with HCHWA

Case No.	Sex	Age at onset	Duration years	Mental symptoms	Epilepsy	Cystatin CSF level
Group I (deceased)						
1	M	20	2.5	2.5 years D1 → D3	no	
2	F	24	(10 days)	coma	no	
3	F	22	3	dysphasia	yes	
4	F	22	5	1 year D1 →	yes	
5	F	27	2.5	>1 year D1 → D3	no	
6	F	26	4.5	0	yes*	
7	M	24	5.5	→ D3	no	1.9
8	F	27	4	2 years D1 → D3	yes	3.8
9	F	25	8	8 years D1 → D3	yes	3.1; 1.7
10	M	20	14	>2 years D1 → D2	no	2
11	M	20	15	12 years D1 → D3	yes	2.9
12	F	26	9.5	8 years D1 → D3	no	
13	F	27	10	>4 years D1 → D3	yes	3
14	F	26	11	>3 years D2 → D3	no	
15	F	26	11.5	>4 years D1 → D3	no	2.1
16	M	25	14.5	>10 years D1 → D2	yes	1.6
17	M	41	>5	>5 years D1 → D3**	no	
Group II (alive)						
18	F	23	3	0	no	2.1
19	F	21	7	dysphasia	no	1.8
20	F	27	2.5	→ D3 → stupor	no	1.4
21	F	32	8	>3.5 years D1 →	yes	2.6
22	F	29	22	16 years D1 → D3 → stupor	yes	2.3

* Involuntary laughing during photic stimulation.
** The case presented with dementia.
Age at onset of symptoms, approximate duration of disease, presence or absence of dementia and epilepsy, and in 12 subjects, the level of cystatin C in the CSF (normal range 4.0–13.6 mg/l). In this group there was a reduction of the cystatin C level below 4 mg/l in all 13 cases where this had been measured. Progression of dementia is indicated with an arrow (→).

known symptoms appeared about 15 years before death (case 11 in fig. 1) while one patient died after the first attack of cerebral haemorrhage (case 2). Of the deceased all but one died before 40 years. This patient presented with dementia which was first noted at the age of 41, initially without any gross neurological symptoms. The mean life span in the group was 32 years. In 9 cases the first EEG, taken after the onset of symptoms, was normal. The last record in 11 cases was severely abnormal and, in the rest, showed a moderate abnormality except in case 10, in which the only available record, taken 9 years after the first symptoms appeared and 4.5 years before death, was normal. Generally the EEG changes were non-specific, consisting of an increase of diffuse slow activity, often asymmetrical. In some cases a general disorganization of the EEG pattern with bilateral loss of alpha activity was seen. In case 2 the only record available was isoelectric, taken one day before death, on the tenth day after the first cerebral haemorrhage. Focal or paroxysmal features were rarely observed in this material.

However, epilepsy or epileptic equivalents were noted in 9 cases. Dementia was noted in 17 cases and dysphasia in additional 2 cases. Only 2 cases were classed as mentally normal. Case 2 died after the first insult, and the patient's only EEG record was taken in terminal coma. Table II shows the relation between EEG abnormality and degree of dementia observed at about the same time. Ten out of 16 cases in group I (deceased) had an EEG recording done during the last year before death, and in group

Table II. Correlation of dementia and EEG abnormality

EEG	Dementia				Total
	D0	D1	D2	D3	
E0	1				1
E1	1	2			3
E2		2		2	4
E3	1		1	11	13
Total	3	4	1	13	21

Case 2 who died after the first attack was excluded. For explanation of symbols, see text. Dysphasia, in cases 3 and 19, was taken as D1. The correlation was significant ($r = 0.65$; $p < 0.01$).

II (alive) all 5 cases had a recent EEG (fig. 3). Case 2, who died on the eleventh day after the first cerebrovascular insult and had an isoelectric record, has been excluded. Case 3 and 19, in whom mild dysphasia was the main symptom, are assigned to class D1. There is a statistically significant positive correlation between the degree of dementia and the degree of EEG abnormality ($r = 0.65$; $p < 0.01$).

Discussion

The uniqueness of this material makes it difficult to obtain a meaningful control group. The age distribution at onset in HCHWA is very different from that of other types of cerebral haemorrhage and cerebrovascular dementia which, like the various other types of dementia, mainly affect older age groups, in which age clearly has an unfavourable effect on the prognosis. Ischaemic stroke in young persons without known amyloid angiopathy has a favourable prognosis with respect to recovery and is rarely recurrent [14], whereas in HCHWA recurrence is the rule. Besides, the present EEG material is collected retrospectively and consequently cannot be taken as a random sample of HCHWA cases. Evidently there is much greater probability that an EEG recording has been done on patients with a long duration of disease and many hospitalizations than on those who have died from the first cerebral insult. It will be noted that there are only 6 males in this group of 22 persons. The reason for this is not clear. The incidence of the disease does not differ significantly between males and females (fig. 1). A correlation between the degree of dementia and EEG abnormality might be expected, as such a correlation has been found in several studies on other types of dementia [18, 25, 32]. The progressive dementia and generalized EEG abnormality must be partly caused by loss or alteration of cerebral substance as a consequence of repeated haemorrhages or infarctions. Even if the material is small it is, however, tempting to speculate that the progressive dementia as well as the EEG abnormality in advanced cases of HCHWA may partly be caused by some mechanism similar to those in other types of cerebral amyloidosis.

The incidence of epilepsy in HCHWA is higher than in other stroke patients, where it is less than 8%, both in series including all ages and young persons only [14, 22]. The reason for the more common occurrence of epilepsy in HCHWA may be related to the fact that most of the patients have had repeated diffuse cerebral infarctions and/or haemorrhages [12].

References

1 Arnason, A.: Apoplexie und ihre Vererbung. Acta psychiat. neurol., suppl. VII (1935).
2 Berger, H.: Über das Elektroenzephalogramm des Menschen. Dritte Mitteilung. Arch. Psychiat. NervKrankh. *94:* 16–60 (1931).
3 Carne, C.A.; Adler, M.W.: Neurological manifestations of human immunodeficiency virus infection. Br. med. J. *293;* 462–463 (1986).
4 Chiofalo, N.; Fuentes, A.; Galvez, S.: Serial EEG findings in 27 cases of Creutzfeldt-Jacob disease. Archs Neurol. *37:* 143–145 (1980).
5 Cohen, D.H.; Feiner, H.; Jensson O.; Frangione, B.: Amyloid fibrin in hereditary cerebral haemorrhage with amylodosis (HCHWA) is related to the gastroenteropancreatic neuroendocrine protein, gamma-trace. J. exp. Med. *158:* 623–628 (1983).
6 Fenton, G.W.: Electrophysiology of Alzheimer's disease. Br. med. Bull. *42:* 29–33 (1986).
7 Frey, T.S.; Sjögren, H.: The electroencephalogram in elderly persons suffering from neuropsychiatric disorders. Acta psychiat. scand. *34:* 438–445 (1959).
8 Gaches, J.: The electroencephalogram in genetic and transmissible dementia. Neurology, Proc. 1st Int. Congr. Neurol., Barcelona 1973, pp. 339–348 (Excerpta Medica, Amsterdam 1973).
9 Ghiso, J.; Jensson, O.; Frangione, B.: Amyloid fibrils in hereditry cerebral haemorrhage with amyloidosis is a varient of gamma-trace (cystatin C). Acta neurol. scand. *73:* 309 (1986).
10 Grubb, A.; Jensson, O.; Gudmundsson, G.; Arnason, A.; Löfberg, H.; Malm, J.: Evidence that abnormal metabolism of gamma-trace is the basic defect in hereditary cerebral haemorrhage with amyloidosis. New Engl. J. Med. *311:* 1547–1549 (1984).
11 Gudmundsson, G.; Hallgrimsson, J.; Jonasson, T.A.; Bjarnason, O.: Hereditary cerebral haemorrhage with amyloidosis. Brain *95:* 387–404 (1972).
12 Gudmundsson, G.; Jensson, O.; Johannesson, G.: Epidemiology and clinical aspects of hereditary cerebral haemorrhage with amyloidosis (HCHWA) in Icelandic families. Acta neurol. scand. *73:* 308–309 (1986).
13 Hachinski, V.C.; Lassen, N.A.; Marshall, J.: Multi-infarct dementia, a cause of mental deterioration in the elderly. Lancet *ii:* 207–210 (1974).
14 Hindfelt, B.; Nilsson, O.: The prognosis of ischemic stroke in young adults. Acta neurol. scand. *55:* 123–130 (1977).
15 Jasper, H.H.: Report of the committee on methods of clinical examination in electroencephalography. Electroenceph. clin. Neurophysiol. *10:* 370–375 (1958).
16 Jensson, O.; Gudmundsson, G.; Arnason, A.; Blöndal, H.; Grubb, A.; Löfberg, H.: Hereditary central nervous system gamma-trace amyloid angiopathy and stroke in Icelandic families; in Glenner et al., Amyloidosis, pp. 789–801 (Plenum Publishing, New York 1986).
17 Johannesson, G.; Brun, A.; Gustafson, L.; Ingvar, D.H.: EEG in presenile dementia related to cerebral blood flow and autopsy findings. Acta neurol. scand. *56:* 89–103 (1977).
18 Johannesson, G.; Hagberg, B.; Gustafson, L.; Ingvar, D.H.: EEG and cognitive impairment in presenile dementia. Acta neurol. scand. *59:* 225–240 (1979).

19   Leperre, J.: Apport de l'EEG a la connaissance de la maladie de Creutzfeldt-Jacob; thesis, Paris (1974).
20   Letemendia, F.; Pampiglione, G.: Clinical and electroencephalographic observations in Alzheimer's disease. J. Neurol. Neurosurg. Psychiat. *21:* 167–172 (1958).
21   Levy, R.M.; Bredesen, D.E.; Rosenblum, M.L.: Neurological manifestations of the acquired immunodeficiency syndrome (AIDS). Experience at UCSF and review of the literature. J. Neurosurg. *62:* 475–495 (1985).
22   Louis, S.; McDowell, F.: Epileptic seizures in non-embolic cerebral infarction. Archs Neurol. *17:* 414–418 (1967).
23   Luyendijk, W.; Bots, G.T.A.M.: Familial incidence of ICH; in Pia, Langmaid, Zierski, Advances in diganosis and therapy, pp. 50–56 (Springer, Berlin 1980).
24   Masters, C.L.; Bayreuther, K.: Amyloidogenic proteins in human central nervous system diseases; in Marrink, van Rijswijk, Amyloidosis (Nijhoff, Dordrecht 1986).
25   Mundy-Castle, A.C.; Hurst, L.A.; Beersteeker, D.M.; Prinsloo, T.: The electroencephalogram in the senile psychoses. Electroenceph. clin. Neurophysiol. *6:* 245–252 (1954).
26   Navia, B.A.; Jordan, B.D.; Price, R.W.: The AIDS dementia complex. 1. Clinical features. Ann. Neurol. *19:* 1517–1524 (1986).
27   Schwab, B.S.: EEG studies and their significance in cerebral vascular disease; in Wright, Cerebral vascular disease, pp. 123–132 (Grune & Stratton, New York 1986).
28   Sishta, S.K.; Troupe, A.; Marszalek, K.S.; Kremer, L.M.: Huntington's chorea: an electroencephalographic and psychometric study. Electroenceph. clin. Neurophysiol. *36:* 387–393 (1974).
29   Stigsby, B.; Jóhannesson, G.; Ingvar, D.H.: Regional EEG analysis and regional cerebral blood flow in Alzheimer's and Pick's disease. Electroenceph. clin. Neurophysiol. *51:* 537–547 (1981).
30   Swain, J.M.: Electroencephalographic abnormalities in presenile atrophy. Neurology *9:* 722–727 (1959).
31   Wattendorf, A.F.; Bots, G.T.A.M.; Went, L.N.; Ednts, L.J.: Familial cerebral amyloid angiopathy presenting as recurrent cerebral haemorrhage. J. neurol. Sci. *55:* 121 (1982).
32   Weiner, H.; Schuster, D.B.: The electroencephalogram in dementia – some preliminary observations and correlations. Electroenceph. clin. Neurophysiol. *8:* 479–488 (1956).

Gudjon Johannesson, MD, Department of Neurology, National Hospital,
University of Iceland, IS–101 Reykjavik (Iceland)

Giannitrapani, Murri (eds.), The EEG of Mental Activities,
pp. 75–93 (Karger, Basel 1988)

Alpha Asymmetry, Hemispheric Specialization and the Problem of Cognitive Dynamics

Stuart Butler

The Medical School, Department of Anatomy, Birmingham, England

Asymmetries in the cranial distribution of the alpha rhythm have been known and discussed for almost as long as the human EEG has been recorded. As early as 1939, Raney [6] ascribed them to cerebral dominance, citing as evidence his finding that the asymmetry occurred in opposite directions in identical twins. By the late 1940s, the tendency for alpha rhythm to be lower in amplitude over the left hemisphere than the right was accepted as a normal feature of the EEG of right-handed people, but there seems to have been no discussion of what caused the effect.

Reports began to appear in the early 1970s which suggested that asymmetry in the amplitude of alpha rhythm was associated with cognitive activity. It was found that the asymmetry appeared during the performance of tasks of a verbal or arithmetic nature [for reviews, see ref. 12–14, 23, 35, 56]. These findings reflected the renewed interest in hemispheric specialization stimulated by the work of Sperry and Bogen on Californian commissurotomy patients. The idea that alpha asymmetry was task specific immediately opened up the prospect of using EEG techniques to probe the lateralization of cognitive processes non-invasively in normal people.

A very large neuropsychological literature has since grown up in which alpha asymmetry is used as a tool to examine the role of left and right hemispheres in a wide variety of mental tasks. Indeed it has been used in some laboratories almost as if it were an alternative to the Wada intracarotid amytal test. But there have been warning signs which seem to indicate that the relationship between conventional measurements of alpha asymmetry and the presumed engagement of lateralized processes is not, after all, a simple one.

In this chapter I shall first consider a number of issues which make it necessary to reappraise, or at least refine, the interpretation of task-related alpha asymmetry. I shall argue that the effect is biased by hemispheric specialization but only to the extent that the experimenter is successful in controlling the subjects' mental activity. It will emerge that factors such as mental set and preferences for particular mental strategies are as important as the type of task in determining alpha asymmetry. Finally I shall argue that the methods usually employed to quantify alpha activity actually conceal what is perhaps the most interesting question of all: the time course of hemispheric activation and its relationship to the dynamics of mental activity.

Asymmetry in the amplitude of alpha activity is only one aspect of the relationship between EEG and mental activity. Asymmetries in coherence, in phase and in power have been described for many regions of the EEG spectrum and appear to be related to the lateralization of mental processes. These effects have been found to vary with individual differences such as gender and psychiatric state which may themselves interact with laterality. For these wider aspects of the subject the reader is referred in the first instance to the pioneering work of Giannitrapani [28–33].

Mental Activity and Alpha Asymmetry

Failures to Replicate
A number of experienced investigators have failed to record asymmetries in the alpha rhythm during activities intended to engage the cognitive specialization of one hemisphere [6, 20, 27, 60, 68; John Shaw, personal communication].

In a long and critical discussion of the problem, Gevins and Schaffer [26] point to methodological weaknesses in published studies and they attribute alpha asymmetry to the unilateral activity of motor systems in right handed tasks. Unfortunately, Gevins and Schaffer [26] did not show that this asymmetry reversed during left-handed activities, nor did they explain how the weaknesses they list might have induced (rather than obscured) EEG asymmetries. The positive findings have been defended by Davidson and Ehrlichman [17], by Galin et al. [24] and by Glass [34], and in a recent test of Gevins' position we have demonstrated that alpha asymmetries are indeed associated with cognitive processing and not with the loading of receptor or motor systems [15].

Although Gevins' rejection of a large and consistent literature is itself unsound, it is obviously puzzling that he and others have been unable to replicate effects which many investigators find remarkably resistant to minor variations in methodology. The effect is evidently more labile or capricious than is desirable in a technique for investigating hemispheric specialization.

The Right Hemisphere

There are very few reports which clearly demonstrate a suppression of alpha rhythm over the right hemisphere during visuo-spatial tasks, or indeed during any form of task which depends upon representational imagery rather than symbolic processing.

This is due in part to the manner in which the asymmetry has been assessed. In many laboratories, it is the custom to compare left-right ratios of alpha power for different tasks and not to contrast the values for individual tasks with some baseline measure [21, 23, 24]. This avoids the problem of defining a baseline, but it does not enable differences in the magnitude of asymmetry to be distinguished from reversals in its direction. Of course, simple left-right differences or ratios for particular tasks are not informative by themselves because systematic variations in skull thickness reduce the amplitude of the EEG over the left hemisphere [11, 52]. It is possible to use the alpha amplitude 'at rest' as a baseline against which to measure changes during task performance. This method runs the risk of systematic bias in the mental activity 'at rest', but it has the advantage of indicating the side of hemispheric activation relative to a single, nominally neutral state. This is therefore the approach we have adopted in our own recent work.

Even when the asymmetry is referred to a resting baseline, few tasks which rely on non-verbal mechanisms induce greater suppression over the right hemisphere than the left. Figure 1 shows the asymmetry relative to a resting baseline during the performance of 8 different tasks by 10 subjects. The first 2 were intended to engage the left hemisphere. The remainder were all designed to activate the right hemisphere: a series of non-verbal discriminations of sounds, tactile shapes, and pictures of faces, together with a 2-dimensional tracking task. Four of the 6 'right hemisphere' tasks produced a large mean asymmetry in the expected direction, but in only one of them did the effect reach statistical significance [57, 58].

In the course of studies over a number of years in our laboratory, we have examined a wide variety of tasks in a search for right hemisphere

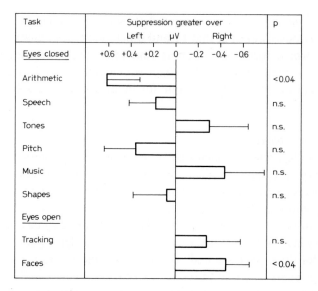

Fig. 1. Mean asymmetry (with standard errors) in the suppression of alpha rhythm in a group of 10 right handed subjects during the performance of tasks designed to engage the cognitive specialization of left and right hemispheres. The recordings were made from left and right occipital regions (01 and 02) with respect to mastoids in common reference.

suppression, including block design, the discrimination of curvature, 3-dimensional tactile puzzles, the discrimination of various types of musical stimuli, evocation of emotional states by music and narrative, and many others, all without effect [1973–1985, unpublished]. Indeed there are no confirmed reports of statistically significant right hemisphere activation relative to a resting baseline on non-covert tasks, with the exception of those involving drawing and the discrimination of faces and facial expression.

It is difficult to maintain that measurements of alpha asymmetry reveal functional lateralization if tasks whose performance is critically dependent upon the right hemisphere are not reliably accompanied by greater suppression over that half of the brain.

Individual Differences in the Lateralization of Language and in Alpha Asymmetry

Although language and other forms of symbolic thinking such as arithmetic [39, 40, 53] are normally dependent on mechanisms resident in the left hemisphere, this is not the case in every individual. Extensive left sided lesions and even left hemispherectomy may do no more than delay the onset of speech if the lesions are sustained early in life [3, 62, 63]. In such cases the neuronal circuits responsible for language must reside in the right hemisphere. About 14% of patients with aphasic disturbances appear to have right hemisphere language [5, 10], and intracarotid amytal reveals a similar figure in epileptic patients [63].

In many of these patients the pattern of cortical localization had probably reorganized in response to longstanding neurological abnormalities, and the incidence of right hemisphere language in the population as a whole is undoubtedly much lower. The importance of excluding patients with early brain damage in assessing normal variation in hemispheric specialization is evident from the work of Rasmussen and Milner [63]. They showed that even among epileptics, right hemisphere language was 4 times as common in patients with early left hemisphere lesions as in those with other or later brain damage.

It is difficult to estimate the incidence of right hemisphere language in the normal population because reliable non-invasive techniques for obtaining this information are not available. For example, estimates based on behavioural methods such as split-field tachistoscopy and dichotic listening may not be free from attentional bias arising from scanning habits or from the effects of unintended cognitive strategies [8]. It is likely that in normal people with no history of birth injury or subsequent brain damage, the incidence of right hemisphere language is in the region of 1%, in both right and left handers. Kimura [49] has reported the incidence of aphasic disturbances in a large sample of more than 500 patients with late-onset lesions, chiefly stroke. Of 244 patients with left-sided lesions, 100 were aphasic. Of 179 with right hemisphere lesions only 2 were aphasic.

The incidence of aphasia was somewhat lower in left handers suggesting some difference in brain organization in this group. Although only 5 of the 40 left handers in the study were aphasic, all of them had left hemisphere lesions. Similarly in a retrospective review of patients studied with carotid amytal by Strauss and Wada [70], right-sided language was almost entirely confined to those with known brain damage in childhood.

If alpha asymmetry provides an index of hemispheric specialization, suppression should therefore be greater over the left hemisphere during verbal and arithmetic tasks in almost all subjects. This is by no means the case. Figure 2 shows the distribution of alpha asymmetry in 145 subjects (healthy undergraduates with no known history of brain damage) examined over a period of several years in our laboratory. The asymmetry is

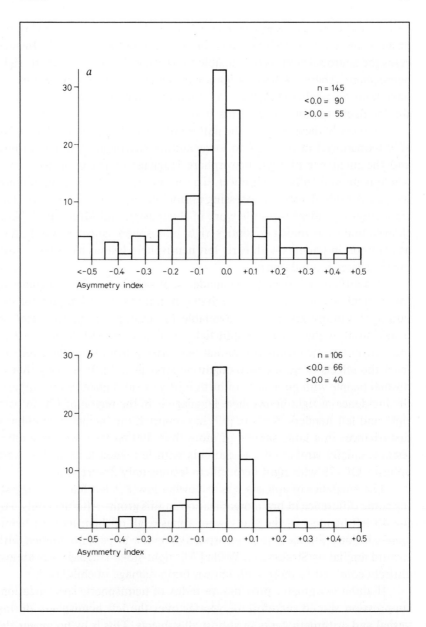

Fig. 2. Asymmetry in the suppression of alpha rhythm during the performance of mental arithmetic by right-handed subjects. Recordings were made from occipital (01 and 02) *(a)* and parietal (P3 and P4) *(b)* electrodes with respect to a common mastoid reference.

calculated against a 'resting' background, i.e. the EEG recorded at the beginning of the experiment while the subject relaxed with eyes closed. In addition, to correct for absolute changes in alpha prevalence, the right-left differences in alpha power are normalized:

$$\text{Asymmetry index} = \frac{(\text{right} - \text{left})}{(\text{right} + \text{left})} \text{ rest} - \frac{(\text{right} - \text{left})}{(\text{right} + \text{left})} \text{ task.}$$

In effect, a negative asymmetry index means that alpha power is suppressed to a greater extent over the left hemisphere during the task.

Figure 2 shows that left hemisphere suppression occurred in two thirds of all subjects during mental arithmetic. These recordings were taken from occipital and parietal regions where such effects are generally most marked. The data for mental arithmetic are presented here because the alpha asymmetry is usually greater and more consistent than that recorded during verbal tasks. Among left-handed subjects, approximately half show left hemisphere suppression during mental arithmetic (fig. 3). These figures clearly do not reflect the incidence of right hemisphere specialization for symbolic processing in the population. Even in left-handed aphasics unselected for the age of onset of brain damage, the incidence of left hemisphere speech is put no lower than 80% [10].

Cognitive Style and the Dynamics of Mental Activity

So far, we have seen that the alpha rhythm becomes asymmetric during the performance of certain tasks, that the direction of this asymmetry appears to reflect the underlying lateralization of brain functions, but that the effect is not consistent enough to reveal hemispheric specialization in a reliable manner. That is surprising, given that electrophysiological techniques monitor brain activity directly. To understand why this may be so it is necessary to consider the structure of mental activity itself in more detail. So far we have simply supposed that particular tasks engage a single hemisphere.

Bogen et al. [7] introduced a new concept into the cerebral dominance literature when they spoke of the 'hemisphericity' of their subjects. This inelegant term was coined to refer to the fact that different individuals employ a variety of cognitive strategies when faced with the same task. This is because a problem can often be tackled in a variety of ways, using for example either representational imagery, or the symbolic processes of

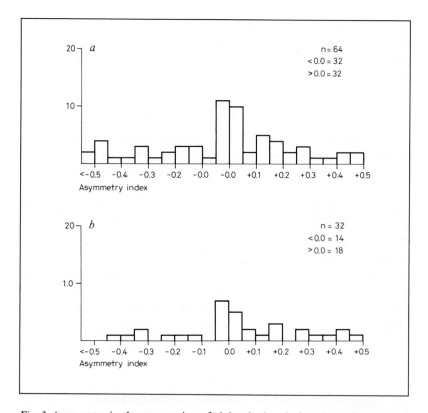

Fig. 3. Asymmetry in the suppression of alpha rhythm during the performance of mental arithmetic by *left-handed* subjects. Recordings were made from occipital (01 and 02) *(a)* and parietal (P3 and P4) *(b)* electrodes with respect to a common mastoid reference.

language or arithmetic. Moreover it appears that people differ in their preference for certain types of cognitive strategy [8]. Such preferences may be regarded as a matter of cognitive style and any given task may therefore be executed using quite different mental and neural processes by different individuals.

In practice the dynamics of mental activity are characterized by a complex interplay of different strategies [16]. For example, mental arithmetic may involve imagery as well as symbolic thinking. The present author is conscious of using imagery for spatial relations, a scratchpad visual memory as well as formal rules of symbol manipulation and rote-learned verbal tables to solve a simple 3 digit mental multiplication. By no means all of these processes can be regarded as 'left hemisphere'. The left hemisphere may be *necessary* for crucial steps within the mental arithmetic and therefore for completion of the task as a whole, but it is probably *not sufficient* to provide all the cognitive mechanisms the individual chooses to employ during the task. The sequence of such processes varies from problem to problem, and undoubtedly the relative importance of cognitive strategies provided by left and right hemispheres varies greatly between individuals.

Even if such complex patterns of cognitive activity are mirrored in the EEG, the methods so far used to study alpha asymmetry would not reveal them. It is customary to perform the spectral analysis on long periods of EEG to ensure that the data are 'representative' of the brain's activity during the task. The asymmetry indices shown in figures 2 and 3 are therefore essentially time averages of the alpha asymmetry over the period occupied by mental arithmetic. Taking such long samples of EEG for analysis only serves to conceal any dynamic changes in hemispheric activation that may accompany an interwoven sequence of cognitive strategies.

Left hemisphere suppression of alpha rhythm in the majority of subjects performing mental arithmetic probably reflects a bias toward the use of strategies provided by this half of the brain. But what of the subjects who exhibit right hemisphere suppression on the same task? These are presumably individuals who make extensive use of spatial strategies during the same task. For them, brief periods of left hemisphere activation during the crucial but transient contributions from this half of the brain are not revealed in the time-averaged alpha asymmetry.

It is not difficult to see why it has proved so difficult to demonstrate a right hemisphere suppression of alpha activity during visuo-spatial tasks. It is hard to exclude verbally mediated intrusions in human thought, particularly under laboratory conditions in which the subjects are given instructions verbally and expect verbal contact with the experimenter at the end. Tasks have seldom been devised and presented to minimize the intrusion of left hemisphere strategies.

If this is correct, we should expect to find that many of the reported EEG asymmetries have as much to do with the balance of cognitive strategies adopted by subjects as with the experimenter's choice of tasks. The tasks are normally selected because the lesion literature indicates that their performance depends crucially on one or the other half of the brain; this ignores the range of supporting strategies which subjects choose to employ.

Evidence for this is provided by the following studies which reveal group differences due to cognitive style and transient effects related to cognitive set.

Cognitive Style as a Function of Gender and Handedness

As we have seen, the incidence of right hemisphere language in the normal population is so small that it leaves little room for group variation in the structural aspects of hemispheric specialization. Yet there are clear indications of group differences in the use and proficiency of verbal and spatial strategies. Verbal skills are acquired earlier and to a higher level by females [9, 25, 45, 47] and some aspects of hand preference are more strongly expressed in females [1, 2, 46]. By contrast, spatial abilities are generally superior in males [41, 50]. Dichotic listening and split-field tachistoscopy reveal asymmetries of performance which appear to be biased by hemispheric specialization but are subject to significant variation as a function of both hand preference and gender [1, 22, 55]. Finally, differences between left and right handers, and between males and females, in the incidence of aphasia after unilateral lesions signify either group differences in cerebral organization or variation in their dependence on particular cognitive strategies [4, 48, 51, 54, 71, 74].

The evidence for sex differences in alpha asymmetry is not consistent. A number of studies have reported that alpha suppression is greater over the left hemisphere in males [31, 36, 64, 65, 72]. But no such differences emerge from a retrospective review of all the data in figure 1 (in which the proportion of males to females is approximately 2:1), nor from a number of studies by others [18, 21, 24, 42–44, 59, 66, 73]. There are no reports of greater left hemisphere suppression in females, in spite of their superiority on behavioural measures of verbal performance.

However Galin et al. [24] reported an interaction between handedness and gender. They found the highest incidence of reversed alpha asymmetry in left-handed females. We have observed a similar interaction in a study of 48 subjects divided into equal groups of males and females, with (FS+) and without (FS–) close left-handed relatives [37]. The findings are summarized in figure 4. The subject's EEG was recorded while at rest, during a mental multiplication task and during a test of face recognition. The time-averaged alpha asymmetries showed suppression over the left hemisphere in FS– females irrespective of task. The presence of left-handedness in the family is marked by a shift away from left hemisphere activation (cf. fig. 2, 3). Right hemisphere activation occurs during the faces task only in male

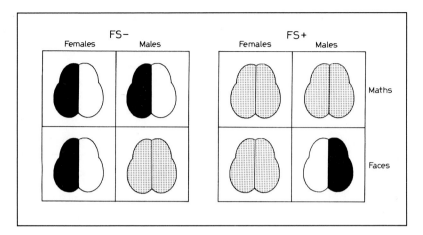

Fig. 4. The pattern of alpha asymmetry in parietal regions in 48 subjects as a function of task, gender and handedness. Stippling indicates that no change occurred in alpha asymmetry relative to the resting baseline. Where a significant change was observed, black shading indicates the hemisphere over which alpha suppression was greater. Subjects with and without left-handed relatives are indicated by FS+ and FS– (FS = familial sinistral).

subjects with left-handed relatives. The data seem to indicate that being female, working on a mathematical task and having no left-handed relatives disposes the individual to prefer strategies dependent upon the left hemisphere. Being male, having left-handed relatives and having to perform a face recognition task encourages greater use of the right hemisphere. Differences in cognitive style therefore must be at least as important as the underlying hemispheric specialization or the nature of the task in determining the direction of alpha asymmetry.

The Effect of Cognitive Set

The phenomenon of 'Einstellung' or 'set' is well known in cognitive psychology. It refers to the bias that may be introduced into perception or cognition by a variety of factors including the manner in which a task is presented, the content of foregoing events or changes in the emotional or motivational state of the subject. Early attempts to investigate the influence of set on alpha asymmetry were inconclusive [19, 67] although serial effects have been clearly demonstrated by Grabow et al. [38].

Two studies from our own laboratory reveal transient but highly significant effects of set on alpha asymmetry. The first was primarily designed

n	Task order			
4	Cartoons	Writing	Drawing	Maths
4	Cartoons	Drawing	Writing	Maths
4	Drawing	Writing	Cartoons	Maths
4	Writing	Drawing	Cartoons	Maths

Fig. 5. Task order in the experiment which revealed set as a serial order effect.

to discover whether the EEG effects could be attributed to asymmetric loading of motor or sensory systems [15, 69]. Subjects had to view cartoons in half the visual field, and to write and to draw with each hand. The tasks were presented in balanced pseudorandom order (fig. 5) and the experiment concluded with a mental arithmetic task, originally included simply as a check that effects we regularly observed were being obtained with new equipment. Figure 6 shows the magnitude of the alpha asymmetries recorded over left and right occipital regions, expressed as asymmetry indices. The histograms marked A are based on recordings from all subjects. In this case it happens that the effects are in the direction that would be expected if the asymmetry simply reflected the lateralization of processes essential for their performance. The evidence for set as a carry over effect emerges if we remove from each analysis the subjects for whom the previous task depended on the opposite hemisphere. When this is done the mean amplitude of the alpha asymmetry increases and the variance decreases. This indicates that subjects tend to perseverate with a particular type of cognitive strategy, or that facilitation of the mechanisms of one hemisphere outlasts the immediate call on them.

This finding prompted us to manipulate cognitive set deliberately in a further experiment. We were particularly concerned about the possible effects of the experimenter as a potential conversant. We therefore measured the alpha asymmetry of 18 subjects while they sat, relaxed with eyes open, in a sound-proofed chamber [11]. For half of the group the recording was first made with the door closed. They were assured that they would be left to relax for several minutes undisturbed. After 3 min the door was

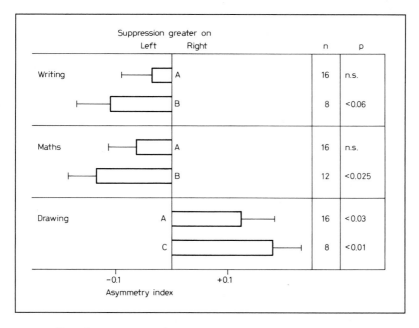

Fig. 6. Effect of the carry-over of set on alpha asymmetry. The histograms labelled A show the mean alpha asymmetry (with standard errors) over all 16 subjects in the study. Those labelled B or C show the mean values for subjects in which maths or writing were not preceded by drawing (B) and drawing was not preceded by writing (C).

opened on the pretext of adjusting an electrode and the measurement repeated, but the chamber door was left open and the experimenter remained in view of the subject. The order of these measurements was reversed for the second half of the group. The power of the alpha rhythm in parietal and occipital regions was remarkably symmetrical while subjects believed they were isolated but it dropped over the left hemisphere when the experimenter was within view and earshot (fig. 7). Since the subject was given no task to perform, the effect appears to be due to some form of social facilitation, presumably a set for verbal communication.

The influence of set on the EEG is important because it supports the hypothesis that alpha asymmetry is primarily a measure of hemispheric activation and only incidentally one of hemispheric specialization. The effects of social facilitation are also important in the light of the failures to replicate task induced alpha asymmetry described earlier. After the first reports of negative findings, we suggest that care needed to be taken to

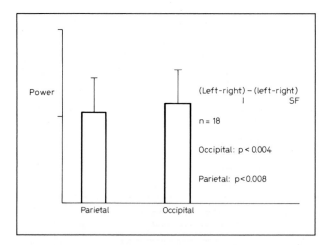

Fig. 7. The effect of isolation, I (subject in sound-proof chamber with door closed) and social facilitation, SF (subject in sound-proof chamber, but door open and experimenter visible). Recordings from 01, 02, P3 and P4 with respect to common mastoid reference. The histograms represent the change in asymmetry of alpha power (arbitrary units) between the two conditions.

ensure that subjects were isolated from the experimenter [14] because the presence of a potential conversant might bias hemispheric activation toward the left to such an extent that nominal task performance would produce no further modulation of alpha power. Many of the early negative findings certainly emanated from open laboratories shared by subject and experimenter. It is not clear from the published reports whether this has always been the case in more recent studies.

The Case for Monitoring the Dynamics of EEG Asymmetry

We have seen that current techniques for studying alpha asymmetries do not provide the same type of information about hemispheric specialization as the effects of unilateral lesions or carotid amytal. The former provides an average measure of left and right activation throughout the execution of a task. Lesion and amytal studies reveal whether a task involves steps which are crucially dependent on one half of the brain.

In retrospect it is remarkable that anyone should have thought to use the average alpha asymmetry over time to measure the lateralization of cerebral functions. An experimenter can set tasks for subjects to perform but has no further control over the cognitive processes which occur. Even before the concept of 'hemisphericity' it should have been clear that no task was likely to exercise the neural mechanisms of a single hemisphere without intrusions from the other side. Task-long epochs of spectral analysis therefore reveal very little about the lateralization of particular cognitive mechanisms. It just happens that if you take a large enough sample, certain tasks (principally arithmetic, reading, writing and face discrimination) change the mix of cognitive strategies enough to produce statistically significant biases in the time-averaged asymmetry. These are not reliable enough to be used as clinical tools for detecting abnormal patterns of hemispheric specialization in individual subjects. Nor do they tell us much about the lateralization of neural mechanisms employed in arithmetic, reading, writing or face recognition because even these activities involve a complex interplay of left and right hemisphere mechanisms, obscured in the time averages.

Alpha asymmetry as it has been measured in the past is therefore not an appropriate tool for investigating the lateralization of cognitive functions. It can only tell us the overall balance of hemispheric usage during particular activities. This may be of value for certain psychological and psychiatric applications, but it has not extended our knowledge of hemispheric specialization. Nor has it established any bridgeheads between cognitive and electrocortical activity.

An understanding of the neural events which underlie on-going mental activity will depend upon the ability to resolve the dynamics of cortical activation in much finer detail. This will require an ability to monitor the rapid switching of hemispheric and regional activation that must take place as different cognitive strategies come into play. This presents a formidable technical problem. In the first instance the problem will be to gain some insight into general patterns of cortical dynamics. The techniques currently available for displaying rapid changes in patterns of cortical activity are somewhat limited. Multichannel compressed spectral arrays and kinematic topograms of the power in individual EEG frequency bands may be helpful. Undoubtedly the greatest difficulty will be to identify specific cognitive processes with particular patterns of electrical activity for as yet we have no independent verification of the fleeting and covert microstructure of mental activity.

Acknowledgements

Much of the work summarized in this chapter was carried out at Birmingham in collaboration with Dr. Alan Glass and our students John Carter, Steve Fisher, Karen Hammond, Megan Griffiths, Pat MacCarthy, Gill MacGrattan, Peter Nava, Ian Pollard, and Alan Stern, with computation assisted by Dr. Roger Flinn.

References

1 Annett, M.: Handedness; in Beaumont, Divided visual field studies of cerebral organisation, pp. 195–215 (Academic Press, London 1982).
2 Annett, M.: Left, right, hand and brain: the right shift theory (Erlbaum, London 1985).
3 Basser, L.S.: Hemiplegia of early onset and the faculty of speech with special reference to the effects of hemispherectomy. Brain 85: 427–460 (1962).
4 Basso, A.; Capitani, E.; Moraschini, S.: Sex differences in recovery from aphasia. Cortex 18: 469–475 (1982).
5 Basso, A.; Capitani, E.; Laiacona, M.; Zanobio, M.E.: Crossed aphasia: one or more syndromes? Cortex 21: 25–45 (1985).
6 Beaumont, J.G.; Mayes, A.R.; Rugg, R.D.: Asymmetry in EEG alpha coherence and power. Effects of task and sex. Electroenceph. clin. Neurophysiol. 45: 393–401 (1978).
7 Bogen, J.E.; DeZure, R.; Tenhouten, W.D.; Marsh, S.F.: The other side of the brain. IV. The A/P ratio. Bull. Los Angeles Neurol. Soc. 37: 49–61 (1972).
8 Bryden, M.P.: Strategy effects in the assessment of hemispheric asymmetry; in Underwood, Strategies of information processing, pp. 117–149 (Academic Press, New York 1978).
9 Bryden, M.P.: Evidence for set-related differences in cerebral organization; in Wittig, Peterson, Sex-related differences in cognitive functioning, pp. 121–139 (Academic Press, New York 1979).
10 Bryden, M.P.; Hecaen, H.; De Agostini, M.: Patterns of cerebral organization. Brain Lang. 20: 249–262 (1983).
11 Butler, S.R.; Fisher, S.; Glass, A.: EEG asymmetry and skull thickness. Electroenceph. clin. Neurophysiol. 63: 79P (1986).
12 Butler, S.R.; Glass, A.: Asymmetries in the alpha rhythm following commissurotomy in man. Electroenceph. clin. Neurophysiol. 34: 728 (1973).
13 Butler, S.R.; Glass, A.: Asymmetries in the electroencephalogram associated with cerebral dominance. Electroenceph. clin. Neurophysiol. 36: 481–491 (1974).
14 Butler, S.R.; Glass, A.: EEG correlates of cerebral dominance; in Reisen, Thompson, Advances in psychobiology, vol. 3, pp. 219–273 (Wiley, New York 1976).
15 Butler, S.R.; Glass, A.: The validity of EEG alpha asymmetry as an index of the lateralisation of human cerebral function; in Papakostopoulos, Butler, Martin, Clinical and experimental neuropsychophysiology, pp. 370–395 (Croom Helm, London 1985).

16   Cohen, G.: Theoretical interpretations of lateral asymmetries; in Beaumont, Divided visual field studies of cerebral organization, pp. 87–111 (Academic Press, London 1982).

17   Davidson, R.J.; Ehrlichman, H.: Lateralised cognitive processes and the electroencephalogram. Science 207: 1005–1006 (1980).

18   Davidson, R.J.; Schwartz, G.E.; Pugash, E.; Bromfield, E.: Sex differences in patterns of EEG asymmetry. Biol. Psychol. 4: 119–138 (1976).

19   Doktor, R.; Bloom, D.M.: Selective lateralization of cognitive style related to occupation as determined by EEG asymmetry. Psychophysiology 14: 385–387 (1977).

20   Donchin, E.; Kutas, M.; McCarthy, G.: Electrocortical indices of hemispheric utilization; in Harnad, Doty, Goldstein, Jaynes, Krauthamer, Lateralization in the nervous system, pp. 339–384 (Academic Press, New York 1977).

21   Ehrlichman, H.; Wiener, M.S.: EEG asymmetry during covert mental activity. Psychophysiology 17: 228–235 (1980).

22   Fairweather, H.: Sex difference: little reason for females to play midfield; in Beaumont, Divided visual field studies of cerebral organization, pp. 147–194 (Academic Press, London 1982).

23   Galin, D.; Ornstein, R.: Lateral specialization of cognitive mode: an EEG Study. Psychophysiology 9: 412–418 (1972).

24   Galin, D.; Ornstein, R.; Herron, J.; Johnstone, J.: Sex and handedness differences in EEG measures of hemispheric specialization. Brain Lang. 16: 19–55 (1982).

25   Gates, A.I.: Sex differences in reading ability. Elementary School J. 61: 431–434 (1961).

26   Gevins, A.; Schaffer, R.: A critical review of electroencephalographic correlates of higher cortical functions. CRC crit. Rev. Bioengng 4: 113–164 (1980).

27   Gevins, A.S.; Zeitlin, G.M.; Doyle, J.C.; Yingling, C.D.; Schaffer, R.E.; Callaway, E.; Yeager, C.L.: Electroencephalogram correlates of higher cortical functions. Science 203: 665–668 (1979).

28   Giannitrapani, D.: EEG phase asymmetries and laterality preference in Clin. Neurophysiol. EEG-EMG, Commun., pp. 301–305 (Verlag der Wiener Medizinischen Akademie, Wien 1965).

29   Giannitrapani, D.: Sex differences in EEG spectra. Electroenceph. clin. Neurophysiol. 37: 434–435 (1974).

30   Giannitrapani, D.: EEG correlates of sex and schizophrenia. Soc. Neurosci. Abstr. 5: 206 (1979).

31   Giannitrapani, D.: Sex differences in the electrophysiology of higher cortical functions. Electroenceph. clin. Neurophysiol. 52: S136 (1981).

32   Giannitrapani, D.: Distribution of EEG power and coherence relating to gender. Neuroscience suppl., 7: S80 (1982).

33   Giannitrapani, D.; Snekhaus, R.: Sex differences in the phase analysis of the human EEG. Electroenceph. clin. Neurophysiol. 23: 589–590 (1967).

34   Glass, A.: Cognitive and EEG asymmetry. Biol. Psychol. 19: 213–217 (1984).

35   Glass, A.; Butler, S.R.: Asymmetries in suppression of alpha rhythm possibly related to cerebral dominance. Electroenceph. clin. Neurophysiol. 34: 729 (1973).

36   Glass, A.; Butler, S.R.; Allen, D.: Sex differences in the functional specialisation of the cerebral hemispheres. Proc. 10th Int. Congr. of Anatomists, Tokyo, p. 204 (Science Council of Japan, Tokyo 1975).

37 Glass, A.; Butler, S.R.; Carter, J.C.: Hemispheric asymmetry of EEG alpha activation: effects of gender and familial handedness. Biol. Psychol. *19:* 169–188 (1984).

38 Grabow, J.D.; Aronson, A.E.; Greene, K.L.; Offord, K.P.: A comparison of EEG alpha activity in the left and right hemispheres by power-spectrum analysis during language and non-language tasks. Electroenceph. clin. Neurophysiol. *47:* 460–472 (1979).

39 Grewel, F.: Acalculia. Brain *75:* 397–407 (1952).

40 Grewel, F.: The acalculias; in Vinken, Bruyn, Handbook of clinical neurology, vol. 4, pp. 181–194 (North-Holland, Amsterdam 1969).

41 Harris, L.J.: Sex differences in spatial ability: possible environmental, genetic and neurological factors; in Kinsbourne, Asymmetrical function of the brain, pp. 405–522 (Cambridge University Press, Cambridge 1978).

42 Haynes, W.O.: Task effect and EEG alpha asymmetry: an analysis of linguistic processing in two modes. Cortex *16:* 95–102 (1980).

43 Haynes, W.O.; Moore, W.H., Jr.: Sentence imagery and recall: an electroencephalographic evaluation of hemispheric processing in males and females. Cortex *17:* 49–62 (1981).

44 Haynes, W.O.; Moore, W.H., Jr.: Recognition and recall: an electroencephalographic investigation of hemispheric alpha asymmetries for males and females on perceptual and retrieval tasks. Percept. Mot. Skills *53:* 283–290 (1981).

45 Herzberg, F.; Lepkin, M.A.: A study of sex differences on the Primary Mental Abilities Test. Educ. Psychol. Measures *14:* 687–689 (1954).

46 Hicks, R.E.; Kinsbourne, M.: Human handedness: a partial cross fostering study. Science *192:* 908–910 (1976).

47 Hutt, C.: Sex differences in human development. Hum. Dev. *15:* 153–170 (1972).

48 Inglis, J.; Ruckman, M.; Lawson, J.S.; MacLean, A.W.; Monga, T.N.: Sex differences in the cognitive effects of unilateral brain damage. Cortex *18:* 257–276 (1982).

49 Kimura, D.: Speech representation in an unbiased sample of left handers. Hum. Neurobiol. *2:* 147–154 (1983).

50 Kimura, D.; Harshman, R.A.: Sex differences in brain organization for verbal and non-verbal functions; in De Vries et al., Progress in brain research, vol. 61, pp. 423–441 (Elsevier, Amsterdam 1984).

51 Landsell, H.: Laterality of verbal intelligence in the brain. Science *135:* 922–923 (1962).

52 Leissner, P.; Lindholm, C.E.; Petersen, I.: Alpha amplitude dependence on skull thickness as measured by ultrasound technique. Electroenceph. clin. Neurophysiol. *29:* 392–399 (1970).

53 Levin, H.S.: The acalculias; in Heilman, Valenstein, Clinical neuropsychology, pp. 128–140 (Oxford University Press, New York 1979).

54 McGlone, J.: Sex differences in human brain organization: a critical survey. Behav. Brain Sci. *3:* 215–227 (1980).

55 McKeever, W.F.; Van Deventer, A.D.: Visual and auditory language processing asymmetries: influence of handedness, familial sinistrality and sex. Cortex *13:* 225–241 (1977).

56 Morgan, A.H.; McDonald, P.J.; MacDonald, H.: Differences in bilateral alpha activity as a function of experimental task, with a note on lateral eye movements and hypnotisability. Neuropsychologia *9:* 459–469 (1971).

57 Nava, P.: EEG correlates of right hemisphere activity; BSc thesis, Birmingham (1974).
58 Nava, P.N.; Butler, S.R.; Glass, A.: Asymmetries of the alpha rhythm associated with functions of the right hemisphere. Electroenceph. clin. Neurophysiol. *43:* 582 (1975).
59 Ornstein, R.E.; Johnstone, J.; Herron, J.; Swencionis, C.: Differential right hemisphere engagement in visuospatial tasks. Neuropsychologia *18:* 49–64 (1980).
60 Provins, K.A.; Cunliffe, P.: The relationship between EEG activity and handedness. Cortex *8:* 136–146 (1972).
61 Raney, E.T.: Brain potentials and lateral dominance in identical twins. J. exp. Psychol. *24:* 21–39 (1939).
62 Rasmussen, T.: Discussion on the current status of cerebral dominance. Res. Publs Ass. Res. nerv. ment. Dis. *42:* 113–115 (1964).
63 Rasmussen, T.; Milner, B.: The role of early left brain injury in determining lateralization of cerebral speech function. Ann. N.Y. Acad. Sci. *229:* 355–369 (1977).
64 Ray, W.J.; Morrell, M.; Fredianai, A.; Tucker, D.M.: Sex differences and lateral specialization of hemispheric functioning. Neuropsychologia *14:* 391–394 (1976).
65 Ray, W.J.; Newcombe, N.; Semon, J.; Cole, P.M.: Spatial abilities, sex differences and EEG functioning. Neuropsychologia *19:* 719–722 (1981).
66 Rebert, C.; Mahoney, R.A.: Functional cerebral asymmetry and performance. III. Reaction time as a function of task, hand, sex and EEG asymmetry. Psychophysiology *15:* 9–16 (1978).
67 Robbins, K.I.; McAdam, R.A.: Interhemispheric alpha asymmetry and imagery mode. Brain Lang. *1:* 189–193 (1974).
68 Rugg, M.D.; Dickens, A.M.J.: Dissociation of alpha and theta activity as a function of verbal and visuospatial tasks. Electroenceph. clin. Neurophysiol. *53:* 201–207 (1982).
69 Stern, A.; Glass, A.; Butler, S.R.: Sensory, motor and cognitive influences on task induced lateral asymmetries in the distribution of alpha rhythm. Electroenceph. clin. Neurophysiol. *52:* 103P (1981).
70 Strauss, E.; Wada, J.: Lateral preferences and cerebral speech dominance. Cortex *19:* 125–130 (1983).
71 Sundet, K.: Sex differences in cognitive impairment following unilateral brain damage. J. clin. exp. Neuropsychol. *8:* 51–61 (1986).
72 Trotman, S.C.A.; Hammond, G.R.: Sex differences in task-dependent EEG asymmetries. Psychophysiology *16:* 429–431 (1979).
73 Tucker, D.M.: Sex differences in hemispheric specialization for synthetic visuospatial functions. Neuropsychologia *14:* 447–454 (1976).
74 Warrington, E.K.; Pratt, R.T.: Language laterality in left handers assessed by unilateral ECT. Neuropsychologia *11:* 423–428 (1973).

Stuart Butler, PhD, Department of Anatomy, The Medical School, Vincent Drive, Birmingham B15 2TJ (England)

Giannitrapani, Murri (eds.), The EEG of Mental Activities,
pp. 94–105 (Karger, Basel 1988)

Hemispheric Asymmetry in the
Perception of Musical Chords:
EEG Laterality and Dichotic Advantage

Pietro San Martini, Rossella Rossi

Department of Psychology, University of Rome, Rome, Italy

The dichotic listening procedure has provided a convenient way of studying hemispheric specialization in the auditory system. Using this procedure, different stimuli presented simultaneously to each ear were lateralized in the hemisphere contralateral to the ear of presentation. Dichotically presented stimuli of linguistic nature, such as words or consonant-vowel syllables, have consistently produced a right-ear advantage reflecting left hemispheric specialization. In contrast, a left-ear advantage has been found for the perception of dichotically, in some cases monaurally, presented musical material such as: melodies [6, 13, 14, 27; Mazzucchi et al., unpublished 1980], chords [4, 7, 8, 10, 17, 21] and musical tones [24]. This supports the generally accepted view that there is some kind of right hemispheric specialization for certain musical functions. In this latter area, however, the available data are less clear-cut since right-ear advantages have been found also for melodies [1, 4, 9, 12] as well as no-ear advantages for chords [8, 10] and for tonal patterns [9].

The general picture outlined above is reflected at the EEG level. Based on the assumption that lateralized processing should result in selective activation of one hemisphere, EEG studies (both of the on-going activity and of evoked potentials) have been carried out to differentiate lateral involvement during the processing of different materials. Although left hemispheric activation has been consistently found for verbal and spatial tasks and for mental arithmetic, attempts to find differential EEG asymmetry during musical tasks have led to conflicting results. Right hemispheric asymmetry has been shown for tasks involving listening to: melodies [15, 20, 26], pieces of music [22], chords [25] and popular songs [11] as well as in singing and whistling [2, 5]. No hemispheric asymmetry has been found for tasks involving: tonal memory testing [3], listening to melodies [16], singing [23], females listening to melodies [22] and whistling a song [2], and musically trained subjects whistling and listening to a familiar song [2, 11]. Left hemispheric asymmetry has been found when humming self-generated melodies [18].

Generally, results of experiments involving musical processing have been shown to be highly dependent on a series of interacting variables such as: the nature of musical material (familiarity, complexity, melodic vs rhythmical vs harmonic), the nature of the task (delayed vs immediate recognition, single vs multiple choice, degree of difficulty) and individual differences (sex, musical skills). The term musical function might be a misleading one since this label applies to a heterogeneous complex of different processes. The majority of the discrepancies found in the literature on this topic can be easily explained if one keeps in mind that lateralization is not dependent upon the material processes per se but on the mode of processing. This in turn can be influenced in a complex manner by the nature of material and task and by individual differences in the preferences of perceptual strategies (analytical-global, serial-parallel).

It therefore may be assumed that, in a study of EEG asymmetry during musical tasks, selection of subjects according to their processing strategies as revealed by the dichotic procedure will result in a reduction of the experimental error and in being more clear cut. The aim of the present study is to verify this assumption in the case of a chord recognition situation. The hypothesis can be specified as follows: (1) there is an asymmetry in EEG activity during processing of chords, and (2) the direction of the asymmetry varies according to the direction of lateralization shown by the subject's performance on a dichotic chord test. The study is divided into 2 separate phases: a dichotic testing session (experiment I) and an EEG session (experiment II).

Experiment I

Subjects

Forty right-handed subjects, 23 males and 17 females with no or low musical competence and between 17 and 30 years of age, participated.

Methods and Materials

Subjects were administered 2 dichotic tests: Gordon's chord test [7] and a syllable test devised by Morra et al. [19]. The latter test of verbal lateralization was added both as a control and to collect data on the relationship between verbal and musical asymmetries.

The chord test, a copy of Gordon's dichotic chord test [7], consisted of 24 dichotic pairs of chords, each followed by a string of 4 binaural chords. The subject sat in a comfortable chair and heard the dichotic pair played through stereo headphones for a duration of 2.5 s. After 1.5 s 4 successive chords were presented binaurally, each for 2.5 s and each separated by 1.5 s. The subject designated which of the binaural chords had been presented dichotically by marking an X with the right hand in the 2 appropriate boxes of an answer sheet. The test, preceded by 4 practice trials, was repeated twice, the second time with headphones rotated between the ears.

The dichotic syllable test followed the same multiple choice paradigm and was administered with the same procedure as the Gordon test. Thirty pairs of stop consonant-vowel syllables were delivered dichotically, each separated by an interval of 5 s. The subject had to mark on an answer sheet which of a string of 6 syllables (pa ta ka ba da ga) had been presented. This test was repeated a second time with headphones rotated between the ears. All stimuli were presented at approximately 70 dB SPL. The entire session lasted about 1 h.

Results

Descriptive and inferential statistics of both dichotic tests are shown in table I. The model used for the analyses of variance is a 2 × 2 (right/left ear, 1st/2nd trial) repeated measures design.

Chord Test

Though the mean score for the left ear was slightly higher than the score for the right ear, the ANOVA did not show any significant advantage of one ear over the other ($F = 1.286$; $p = 0.262$): 18 of the 40 subjects showed a right ear advantage (R > L), 21 a left ear advantage (L > R) and 1 no advantage (L = R). Nearly half of the subjects (19 of 40) scored below the level of chance guessing according to the following criterion (employed by Gordon [8]): the subject had to attain on the average a total (L + R) score of 29 or more ($p < 0.06$, binomial test, one-tailed) or one ear score (L or R) of 17 or more ($p < 0.06$, binomial test, one-tailed). These results are in agreement with Gordon's studies which found on the average no ear advantage in musically uneducated subjects, a similar proportion of chance level scores and slightly higher mean scores [7, 8].

Syllable Test

The analysis of variance yielded a significant main effect of ear ($F = 9.147$; $p = 0.004$) as well as of trial repetition ($F = 32.641$; $p < 0.001$), showing the expected right ear advantage and a practice effect. Correlations between syllable and chord test were all nonsignificant and near zero level.

Table I. Results of the dichotic tests. Mean number of correct responses (standard deviation), F values for the effects of ear and of trial repetition and associated p values (n = 40)

	Chord test		Syllable test	
	right ear	left ear	right ear	left ear
1st trial	13.42 (2.96)	14.00 (3.06)	18.47 (3.23)	16.92 (2.98)
2nd trial	13.47 (2.87)	14.02 (3.10)	20.60 (3.15)	18.95 (3.77)
Mean	13.45	14.01	19.53	17.93
	$F(ear) = 1.286; p = 0.262$		$F(ear) = 9.147; p = 0.004$	
	$F(trial) = 0.009$		$F(trial) = 32.641; p < 0.001$	

Table II. Laterality scores (L–R/L+R* 100) to the chord test of the subjects of the EEG experiment. In parentheses the laterality scores of the syllable test

Left ear lateralyzers	Right ear lateralyzers
27.05 (11.30)	–23.70 (–48.55)
25.55 (–6.85)	–21.45 (–5.01)
20.95 (0.00)	–18.05 (1.95)
11.55 (1.65)	–12.45 (2.7)
10.35 (–1.35)	–6.7 (–15.25)
11.30 (–2.50)	

Experiment II

Subjects

For the EEG experiment 2 groups of 6 subjects were selected. They showed, respectively, the highest and lowest laterality scores (L – R/L + R) for the dichotic chord test. The laterality scores had to be directionally consistent across both presentations of the test and the subject's performance had to be above chance guessing according to the aforementioned criterion. Since one of the right-ear lateralizers abandoned the experiment for personal reasons, 6 subjects (4 females, 2 males) remained in the group of left-ear lateralizers and 5 subjects (1 female, 4 males) in the group of right-ear lateralizers. As may be seen from table II, the laterality scores obtained by our experimental subjects in the chord test were unrelated to the laterality scores of the verbal test.

EEG Recording and Analysis

Subjects were seated in a reclining chair fitted with an adjustable neck rest in a dimly lit sound-proof cubicle. The EEG was recorded from 2 symmetrical parietal derivations with the exploring electrodes placed on P_3 and P_4 and common reference on C_z (international 10–20 system). Time constant was 0.3 s. The 2 polygraph channels were calibrated to 1 V output peak to peak for a 100-µV square wave signal. The traces were fed into a spectral Fourier analyser working on 8-second epochs (resolution: 0.5 Hz, sampling rate 128 points/s). Power spectra of artifact-free periodograms were calculated in the range of 1 and 32 Hz. For the purpose of the subsequent statistical analysis only the summed energy content of the total band (1–32 Hz) and of the alpha band (8–13 Hz) have been considered.

Procedure and Stimulus Conditions

The first problem to be solved in designing the experiment was the selection of a baseline or reference against which to measure the EEG asymmetry. The most obvious one, the resting condition, has been rightly criticized as being largely uncontrolled. We decided therefore to include, as control conditions, several tasks supposedly involving different levels of EEG asymmetry according to the following schedule: (1) Condition B (baseline): after some minutes of adaptation, the resting EEG was recorded for 2 min. (2) Condition M (passive listening to music): the subject was invited to listen to a section of a concert for piano and orchestra (drawn from the sound track of a movie unknown to all subjects), lasting 4 min. (3) Condition CH (passive listening to chords): the subject was invited to listen to 4 successive series of chords. Each series consisted of: one chord (2 s), an interval (2 s) and a string of 4 chords in a run, each lasting 2 s. The chords, originally produced by an electronic organ, consisted of the fundamental, third, fifth and octave, the fundamental being in a range of an octave around middle C. SPL was the same as in the dichotic test (70 dB). (4) Condition M+ (listening to music with recognition task): the subject was invited to listen to the same musical piece as in condition M but was instructed to notice, and later report, how many times the piano joined the orchestra (which happened only once). (5) Condition CH+ (listening to chords with recognition task): the subject was presented with the same material as in condition CH but was instructed to report at the end of each series whether the first chord appeared in the following string of 4 chords. (6) Condition MC (mental calculation): the subject was requested to mentally multiply number 2 by 2, the result again by 2, and so on, until stopped by the experimenter (approximately after 1 min) and asked to report the result.

All stimuli were tape-recorded and delivered through a loudspeaker placed 2 m in front of the subject. All instructions were given by the experimenter just before each trial. The subjects were requested to keep their eyes shut during all conditions and to open them again when the recording was interrupted in order to be given the instructions. The entire EEG session lasted approximately 25 min (including intervals to give instructions).

To summarize, the experimental schedule was the following: baseline (B, 2 min); passive listening to music (M, 4 min); passive listening to chords (CH, 4 min); recognition task of music (M+, 4 min), of chords (CH+, 4 min); and mental calculation (MC, 1 min).

In the control conditions (B, M, M+ and MC) the EEG was continuously sampled by the spectral analyzer. In the experimental conditions (CH, CH+) the tracing was sampled only during the presentation of the strings of chords.

Results

The most common way of analyzing laterality effects in the EEG is through laterality indexes (L – R/L + R), but since these can be the outcome of changes in the absolute level of either or both hemispheres an analysis of within hemisphere effects is also of interest. The data, therefore, have been analyzed both in terms of ratio scores and in terms of within-hemisphere changes.

Effects of the Experimental Variables on the Laterality Index

Mean values and standard errors of laterality scores (L – R/L + R* 100) for the total- and alpha-band power in our experimental condition are depicted in figure 1a and b.

The analysis of variance (ANOVA repeated measures design) of the total power ratio scores showed a significant main effect of the experimental condition (F = 3.166; p = 0.014). Further breakdown of the ANOVA by a split-plot design (table IIIa) to look for interaction effects with lateralization to Gordon test showed no differences between right and left ear lateralizers in the dichotic test (F = 0.509) and no interaction between experimental condition and ear advantage (F = 0.163).

Table III. Summary of the analyses of variance of the laterality scores (L–R/L+R* 100) based (a) on total EEG power (0.1–32 Hz) and (b) on alpha power (8–13 Hz). Split-plot design

Source	SS	DF	MS	F	p
(a) Total power					
Dichotic adv.	704.782	1	704.782	0.509	
Error	12,455.956	9	1,383.995		
Condition	1,858.984	5	371.796	2.858	0.025
Adv.* cond.	106.252	5	21.250	0.163	
Error	5,853.078	45	130.068		
(b) Alpha power					
Dichotic adv.	1,630.278	1	1,630.278	0.956	
Error	15,332.334	9	1,703.278		
Condition	1,389.963	5	277.992	1.282	0.287
Adv.* cond.	321.292	5	64.258	0.296	
Error	9,750.870	45	216.686		

As shown by Duncan's multiple range test for a posteriori comparisons (rejection level: $p < 0.05$) the main effect of the experimental conditions was due (a) to the difference between MC on one side and M, M+ and B on the other; (b) to the difference between CH+ and B. In other words, regardless of the laterality exhibited in the Gordon test by our subjects, condition MC showed differential left hemispheric activation vs M, M+ and B; CH did not differ significantly from any other condition; and CH+ induced a left side shift in activation only with reference to the baseline level. Such main effect of experimental conditions failed to reach significance ($F = 1.457$; $p = 0.219$; repeated measures design) in the alpha band despite an apparent similarity of the pattern of means. The effects of ear laterality and of interaction were also not significant (table IIIb).

Within Hemisphere Effects of the Experimental Variables on the Raw Power Values of the EEG

Means and standard errors of the power values of the right and left derivations of the EEG are depicted in figure 2a (total band power) and 2b (alpha band power).

The analysis of variance (repeated measures design; table IVa, b) showed a significant main effect of the experimental conditions only in the left hemisphere, both for the alpha band ($F = 2.870$; $p = 0.023$) and for the total band ($F = 3.137$; $p = 0.015$). Further breakdown of the ANOVAS by a split-plot model to look in the dichotic test for interaction effects with lateralization showed no differences between right and left hemispheric lateralizers (F values ranging from 0.002 and 0.211) and no interaction between experimental conditions and lateralization (F values ranging from 0.144 and 1.273).

Fig. 1. Mean values and standard errors of the *laterality index* of the EEG (left − right/left + right *100) shown by right ear lateralizers (REL) and left ear lateralizers (LEL) to Gordon's dichotic test as a function of the experimental condition. *a* Laterality index calculated on the basis of the total power of the EEG (1–32 Hz). *b* Laterality index calculated on the basis of the alpha power of the EEG (8–13 Hz). Conditions: B = baseline; M = music (passive condition); CH = chords (passive condition); M+ = music (recognition task); CH+ = chords (recognition task); MC = mental calculation.

Fig. 2. Mean values and standard errors of the *EEG power* of the right (RH) and left (LH) hemisphere as a function of the experimental condition. *a* Values of the total power of the EEG (1–32 Hz). *b* Values of the alpha band power of the EEG (8–13 Hz). Conditions: B = baseline; M = music (passive condition); CH = chords (passive condition); M+ = music (recognition task); CH+ = chords (recognition task); MC = mental calculation.

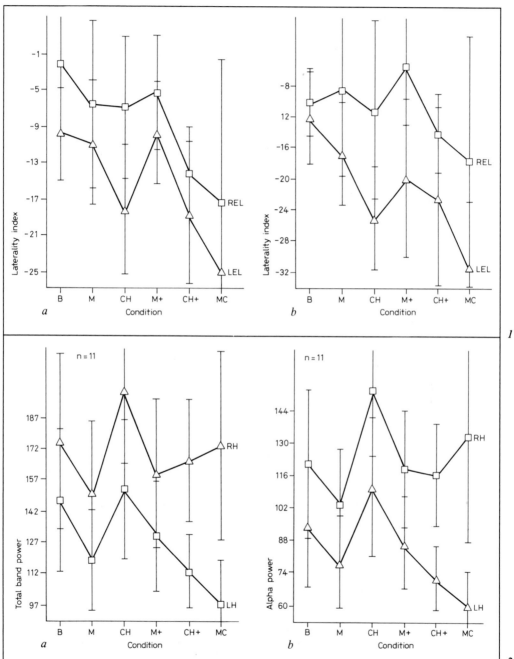

Table IV. Summary of the analyses of variance of the raw power values of the right and left derivations of the EEG. (a) Analyses performed on the total band values (0.1–32 Hz); (b) analyses performed on the alpha band values (8–13 Hz). Repeated measures design

Source	SS	DF	MS	F	p
(a) Total band					
Right hemisphere					
Subjects	748,358.756	10			
Condition	16,021.346	5	3,204.269	0.875	
Error	182,910.150	50	3,658.203		
Left hemisphere					
Subjects	400,222.786	10			
Condition	24,124.121	5	4,824.824	3.137	0.015
Error	76,881.211	50	1,537.624		
(b) Alpha band					
Right hemisphere					
Subjects	392,253.604	10			
Condition	15,491.590	5	3,098.318	0.716	
Error	216,082.575	50	4,321.651		
Left hemisphere					
Subjects	242,379.757	10			
Condition	17,570.802	5	3,514.160	2.870	0.023
Error	61,217.697	50	1,224.353		

Duncan's multiple range test (rejection level: $p < 0.05$) showed that the main effect of the experimental conditions on the left hemisphere was due to the difference between MC on one side and B and CH on the other as well as to the difference between CH+ and CH. In other words, while in the right EEG derivation there was no consistent effect of the experimental condition, in the left EEG derivation our subjects showed a higher level of activation during mental calculation versus both baseline and passive listening to chords and a higher level of activation in the chord recognition condition than in the passive listening to chords condition.

Summary of the EEG Results

(a) On the whole the experimental conditions affected significantly only the left EEG derivation. No mean change in the right derivation was statistically significant.

(b) Ear advantage to the dichotic chord test was not a significant source of variance, neither in terms of laterality index nor in terms of within hemisphere changes.

(c) Processing of chords: the analysis of the laterality indexes showed a left side shift in activation (with reference to the baseline only) occurring when subjects were engaged in the recognition task, whereas passive listening to chords did not differ significantly from any of the other conditions. The analysis of the raw power values showed a higher involvement of the left hemisphere during the recognition task than during passive listening.

(d) Processing of music: as shown by the laterality index, processing of music, both with and without recognition task, differed significantly versus mental calculation, but not versus any of the other conditions. In terms of within hemisphere changes, M and M+ did not differ significantly from any other condition.

(e) Mental calculation produced a left-side shift of the laterality index versus B, M and M+. In terms of within hemisphere effects this condition induced an attenuation of power of the left derivation compared to baseline and passive listening to chords.

Discussion

The present results give evidence of a moderate degree of EEG power asymmetry favoring the left hemisphere during a chord recognition task but fail to support the hypothesis that individual differences of ear advantage in a dichotic chord test significantly affect the EEG measure.

The dependence of EEG asymmetry on the task assigned rather than on the material presented per se is confirmed in the case of musical chord processing. Evidence of differential (left hemisphere) involvement during the presentation of chords was obtained only when subjects were engaged in a multiple choice recognition task, not when they were passively listening to the same material. This shift in activation, similar to that induced by mental calculation, is probably interpretable in terms of selective left hemispheric involvement in the analytic processing mode. These effects of the task did not appear when subjects were instructed to remember and later report the number of piano episodes of an orchestral piece of music. This can be possibly accounted for by the low level of difficulty of this task as opposed to the multiple choice recognition task adopted in the case of chords. An alternative explanation may be in terms of different perceptual strategies evoked by music itself as opposed to an 'abstract' portion of it such as chordal material.

The failure to demonstrate a significant effect of the dichotic chord test results on EEG asymmetry is interpretable in at least 2, not mutually exlusive, ways. (1) In spite of the apparent similarity of the stimulus conditions (same sequence of chords, same recognition task) the very nature of the observations is entirely different. While the variations in asymmetry picked up by the EEG concern an ongoing process which takes place during the entire binaural presentation of the chordal material, the ear advantage picked up by the dichotic test might be due mostly to the early stage of the perceptual process when the storage of the dichotic stimulus takes place. (2) The encouraging data available in the literature on EEG asymmetry during verbal and arithmetical tasks cannot be generalized to the assumption that any lateralization in perceptual processing should express itself in the level of EEG activity, since hemispheric advantage can be the result of processes not monotonically related to cortical arousal.

Concerning points 1 and 2, further information may be sought by modifying the experimental paradigm in order to allow the simultaneous investigation both of the ongoing EEG activity and of the AEP triggered by the dichotic and binaural chords.

References

1   Bever, T.G.; Chiarello, R.J.: Cerebral dominance in musicians and nonmusicians, Science 185: 537–539 (1974).
2   Davidson, R.J.; Schwartz, G.E.: The influence of musical training on patterns of EEG asymmetry during musical and non-musical self-generation tasks. Psychophysiology 14: 58–63 (1977).
3   Doyle, J.C.; Ornstein, R.; Galin, D.: Lateral specialization of cognitive mode: II. EEG Frequency Analysis. Psychophysiology 11: 567–578 (1974).
4   Gaede, S.E.; Parsons, O.A.; Bertera, J.H.: Hemispheric differences in music perception: aptitude vs experience. Neuropsychologia 16: 369–373 (1978).
5   Galin, D.; Ornstein, R.; Herron, J.; Johnstone, J.: Sex and handedness differences in EEG measures of hemispheric specialization. Brain Lang. 16: 19–55 (1982).
6   Goodglass, H.; Calderon, M.: Parallel processing of verbal and musical stimuli in right and left hemispheres. Neuropsychologia 15: 397–407 (1977).
7   Gordon, H.W.: Hemispheric asymmetries in the perception of musical chords. Cortex 6: 387–398 (1970).
8   Gordon, H.W.: Hemispheric asymmetry for dichotically-presented chords in musicians and non-musicians, males and females. Acta psychol. 42: 383–395 (1978).
9   Gordon, H.W.: Left hemisphere dominance for rhythmic elements in dichotically-presented melodies. Cortex 14: 58–70 (1978).

10 Gordon, H.W.: Degree of ear asymmetries for perception of dichotic chords and for illusory chord localization in musicians of different levels of competence. J. exp. Psychol. 6: 516–527 (1980).

11 Hirshkowitz, M.; Earle, J.; Paley, B.: EEG alpha asymmetry in musicians and non-musicians: a study of hemispheric specialization. Neuropsychologia 16: 125–128 (1978).

12 Johnson, P.R.: Dichotically stimulated ear differences in musicians and nonmusicians. Cortex 13: 385–389 (1977).

13 Kimura, D.: Left-right differences in the perception of melodies. Q. J exp. Psychol. 16: 355–358 (1964).

14 Kimura, D.: Functional asymmetry of the brain in dichotic listening. Cortex 3: 168–178 (1967).

15 McKee, G.; Humphrey, B.; McAdam, D.V.: Scaled lateralization of alpha activity during linguistic and musical tasks. Psychophysiology 10: 441–442 (1973).

16 Moore, W.H., Jr.: Alpha hemispheric asymmetry of males and females on verbal and nonverbal tasks: some preliminary results. Cortex 15: 321–326 (1979).

17 Morais, J.; Peretz, I.; Gudanski, M.: Ear asymmetry for chord recognition in musicians and nonmusicians. Neuropsychologia 20: 351–354 (1982).

18 Morgan, A.H.; Macdonald, H.; Hilgard E.R.: EEG alpha: lateral asymmetry related to task and hypnotizability. Psychophysiology 11: 275–282 (1974).

19 Morra, B.; Martini, A.; Cornacchia, L.; Tobey Cullen, F.; Miller, M.: Dichotic performance of Italian subjects tested with English and Italian stopconsonant-vowel stimuli. Audiology 22: 167–171 (1983).

20 Osborne, K.; Gale, A.: Bilateral EEG differentiation of stimuli. Biol. Psychol. 4: 185–196 (1976).

21 Peretz, I.; Morais, J.: A left ear advantage for chords in non-musicians. Percept. Mot. Skills 49: 957–958 (1979).

22 Ray, W.J.; Morell, M.; Frediani, W.: Sex differences and lateral specialization of hemispheric functioning. Neuropsychologia 14: 391–394 (1976).

23 Schwartz, G.E.; Davidson, R.J.; Maer, F.; Broomfield, E.: Patterns of hemispheric dominance in musical, emotional, verbal and spatial tasks (Abstract). Psychophysiology 4: 227 (1974).

24 Sidtis, J.J.; Bryden, M.P.: Asymmetrical perception of language and music: evidence for independent processing strategies. Neuropsychologia 16: 627–632 (1978).

25 Taub, J.M.; Tanguay, P.E.; Doubleday, C.: Clarckson, D.; Remington, R.: Hemisphere and ear asymmetry in the auditory evoked response to musical chord stimuli. Physiol. Psychol. 4: 11–17 (1976).

26 Thomas, D.G.; Shucard, D.W.: The use of a control or baseline condition in electrophysiological studies of hemispheric specialization of function. Electroenceph. clin. Neurophysiol. 55: 575–579 (1983).

27 Zatorre, R.J.: Recognition of dichotic melodies by musicians and nonmusicians. Neuropsychologia 17: 607–617 (1979).

Pietro San Martini, MD, Dipartimento di Psicologia, Università di Roma,
Via degli Apuli 8, I-00186 Roma (Italy)

Giannitrapani, Murri (eds.), The EEG of Mental Activities,
pp. 106–118 (Karger, Basel 1988)

EEG Correlates of Language Impairment in Left Brain-Lesioned Patients

Luigi Murri [a], *Enrica Bonanni* [a], *Roberto Massetani* [a], *Carlo Navona* [b], *Franco Denoth* [b, 1]

[a] Clinical Neurophysiology, Department of Neurology, University of Pisa;
[b] Institute Elaboration of Information, CNR, Pisa, Italy

The considerable amount of information collected over the last 30 years on the complementary specialization of the 2 cerebral hemispheres [see ref. 53] gradually strengthened the hypothesis that the EEG might reveal a different involvement of the 2 hemispheres in processing particular cognitive tasks. With the pioneering work of Galin et al. [14, 15] and Morgan et al. [42], it was found that the different alpha rhythm decrease in the 2 hemispheres depended on the type of task performed. Consequently, the long-standing observation that both verbal and nonverbal mental activities have an alpha rhythm depression as their electrophysiological correlate [1] became specific and significant.

These observations were made possible by the application of automatic signal processing techniques, clearly far less restrictive than visual EEG assessment. Subsequently, a number of studies exploiting these techniques confirmed that a reduction in the EEG signal (generally integrated amplitude or total power associated with the single frequency bands especially alpha) on the left during performance of verbal tasks and on the right during nonverbal tasks is frequent in normal right-handed subjects [see ref. 17]. The study carried out by Butler and Glass [7], using such methods on split-brain patients whose language areas had been investi-

[1] We would like to thank Dr. Monica Mazzoni for performing reaction times and Mr. Giancarlo Santerini for technical assistance.

gated with Wada test, appeared as a further confirmation of the validity of the methodology.

This task-dependent EEG asymmetry therefore indicates that the reduced amplitude and rhythmicity of the alpha band on the left, often visually detectable under rest conditions, cannot be related to a static situation such as handedness, as previously hypothesized by Raney [49] in 1939 though data both supporting this hypothesis [8, 21] and contrasting it [23, 48] were subsequently reported. Similarly, it does not seem likely that this asymmetry depends on anatomic factors, such as bone thickness [36] or the different size of homologous brain areas [37, 55].

As a consequence, the EEG began to be included among a variety of methods applied to the study of the cerebral lateralization of higher cognitive functions in man. It appears more suitable, in fact, than methods such as dichotic listening, tachistoscopic viewing, ERPs and others, as it can be used with natural cognitive tasks which require more than a few milliseconds for information processing. Moreover, this technique allows the study of the different brain regions involved in a task, and can be used even without the collaboration of the subject.

The study of variations in task-dependent EEG asymmetry is founded on 2 suppositions, one electrophysiological and the other neuropsychological. The first is that mental activity is accompanied by a reduction in the signal (usually in the alpha band), and that when this occurs asymmetrically during a cognitive process, it indicates differences in hemispheric involvement in the performance of the particular task. These variations are relative in that signals from both hemispheres will be modified simultaneously but asymmetrically. Moreover, when the asymmetry trend is observed in the single epochs, through time, the variations are seen to fluctuate but show a preference for one side or the other when mean epoch values are considered.

The second supposition is that in right-handed subjects, verbal and analytical-type activities (e.g. reading, writing, classifying, etc.) mainly involve the left hemisphere, whereas tasks of a nonverbal, spatial, holistic and musical type imply a prevalent right hemisphere involvement, independent from differences among these individual tasks [22].

Without doubt, there are electrophysiological difficulties, clearly identified by Donchin et al. [10], linked to differences in the methods used for data collection and quantification. There is also the question of the way in which a task is executed. In our experience, nonmotor auditory tasks have the advantage of reducing movement artifacts which can hinder a correct assessment of EEG data, as often happens with visuomotor tasks, though the latter allow the operator to check that the task is performed properly.

Finally, there have been some discrepancies in interpretations [19, 20] and contradictory data, particularly in regard to nonverbal tasks, suggesting that EEG variations may depend on other factors such as the stimulus characteristics, task difficulty, strategy adopted, individual skill [13, 16, 24, 29, 40, 47, 51, 56]. In this typically interdisciplinary field, therefore, there is the risk of oversimplifying certain aspects of the problem, either accepting a superficial dichotomy between verbal and nonverbal tasks and left and right hemispheres or holding that EEG variations are always cognitive-dependent.

As well as in normal subjects, the study of task-dependent EEG asymmetry has found a number of applications in psychiatric disorders [see ref. 27], but so far it has been little used in investigations on organic brain disease. This scarce interest is surprising, all the more so if we consider that the 19th century findings of Dax and Broca in brain-lesioned patients provided the foundations for the knowledge that the cerebral hemispheres are not functionally identical, and that later data concerning hemispheric specialization emerged from studies on patients with primitive or surgical cerebral lesions [41].

The data obtained from normal subjects suggest that this EEG technique is a valid method for investigating cognitive process deficits in language in brain-lesioned patients. The present study considered 2 extreme conditions of lesions in the left hemisphere. The first occurred in patients who, as a result of acute and extensive lesions in the left hemisphere, presented very severe language comprehension disorders. The second group consisted of temporal lobe epileptics with left EEG focus and without clinically detectable language disorders. Numerous neuropsychological findings indicate that these patients have verbal function deficits, but it is not clear whether or not they depend on the brain lesion and its extent.

Another technique considered valid for the evaluation of hemispheric lateralization, dichotic listening, has shown that results differ among epileptics studied according to whether or not there is evidence of macroscopic lesion of the temporal lobe [39]. The study of reaction times in symptomatic focal seizure patients has also provided different data depending on the extent of the damaged brain structure [5]. In order to exclude these variables, the epileptic patients considered in this study did not have CT-scan-detectable macroscopic lesions.

Material and Method

Twenty-six of the patients studied (14 males and 12 females, age range 62–75 years) were affected by right hemiplegia following acute left-brain lesions caused by supratentorial unilateral infarction as shown by CT scan. Fourteen of these patients had receptive or global aphasia, and 12 showed no language disorders. The shortened version of the Token test [9] showed that the aphasia was very severe in all 14 patients. EEG recordings were effected one week after the ictus, while the patients were being treated with dexamethasone phosphate and or hypertonic solutions.

An additional sample of 14 cases (9 males and 5 females, age range 16–50 years) were all outpatients attending the Epilepsy Centre and had a diagnosis of temporal epilepsy. Other selection criteria were: complex partial seizures without secondary generalization; EEG alterations in left temporal or frontotemporal regions; normal CT scan; absence of other neurological disorders and of psychiatric case history. The patients were all under treatment with various doses of anticonvulsive drugs (phenobarbital, carbamazepine, phenytoin) at the time of the EEG recordings. Serum drug levels were measured within 5 days of the EEG and proved within the therapeutic range in all cases. The level of vigilance in these patients was evaluated by measuring simple visuomotor reaction times.

The control group consisted of 13 normal adult males, all right-handed. In both normal and epileptic patients, handedness was tested using Oldfield's [46] questionnaire, while for patients with acute left hemisphere lesions the evaluation was based on what the patient – or his family in the case of aphasic patients – reported.

During the EEG recording, auditory stimuli were applied through earphones at a comfortable listening level of 60 dB. According to the protocol, the sessions were divided into 4 phases: (1) white noise (WN), considered as neutral baseline condition; (2) meaningful verbal stimulus consisting of listening to an article of general interest; (3) nonverbal stimulus consisting of a passage of classical music (Vivaldi), as numerous data indicate that listening to music involves mainly the right hemisphere [6, 33]; (4) nonmeaningful stimulus consisting of listening to the same article as in (2) read in an unknown foreign language (Finnish dialect). Both control subjects and patients, excluding the aphasics, were instructed to listen carefully to all stimuli, whether comprehensible or not. To verify that they were actively engaged in these tasks, several questions were asked at the end of each stimulus, concerning content in the case of the verbal stimulus, type of music and instruments used in the case of the musical stimulus, and whether anything of the foreign language task had been comprehensible. Each stimulus condition lasted 3 min, with a brief interval between phases to allow for questioning.

EEG activity was recorded from P3, P4, O1 and O2 using intrahemispheric bipolar linkages (P4–O2 and P3–O1). The interelectrode distance was measured carefully to ensure symmetry, and electrode impedance was below 5,000 Ω. The EEG signal was recorded simultaneously on paper (OTE 18-d) and on magnetic tape (Philips Analog-14) to perform automatic off-line analysis. Epochs were of 5 s duration and only artifact-free segments were analyzed. The EEG signals were filtered between 0.25 and 35.0 Hz, digitized at a rate of 102.4 samples per second and processed with an HP 2113/B computer connected to an FFA HP5451/C system. The digital filter used to select each band and total power was a rectangular window in the frequency domain. EEG activity was analyzed according to the following band assignment: total power (1.2–30.0 Hz); delta (1.2–

2.8 Hz); theta-1 (3.0–4.6 Hz); theta-2 (4.8–7.8 Hz); alpha (8.0–12.8 Hz); beta-1 (13.0–19.8 Hz); beta-2 (20.0–30.0 Hz).

In order to compare the EEG of patients with acute cerebral lesions – and thus observe slow elements particularly on the left – with that of the normal subjects, a right/left index was used. The right/left index is the difference between the logarithmic transforms of verbal/musical ratio on the right and that on the left. On the basis of the hypothesis that the left side is predominantly involved in verbal tasks in right-handed subjects, giving a lower EEG signal power, the log verbal/musical ratio on the left will be less than zero. Similarly, the right side should show a relatively lower power during musical tasks with respect to verbal ones, so that the log verbal/musical ratio will be greater than zero on the right.

The subsequent index – log of verbal/musical ratio (right/left) – should prove higher if there is an evident asymmetry between the two hemispheres during a verbal task, while if the asymmetry is only slight or if both tasks provoke the same asymmetry, the value will be close to zero. The index will be negative if the usual verbal task-dependent asymmetry is not observed. The verbal task was also compared with white noise and with the unknown foreign language using same formula.

Table I. Mean verbal/musical and verbal/foreign language index values (± SEM) of total power (TP) and power associated with single frequency bands in normals, aphasic and nonaphasic patients

	TP	Delta	Theta-1	Theta-2	Alpha	Beta-1	Beta-2
Verbal/musical index							
Normals	0.080	0.058	−0.013	0.083	0.130	0.058	0.051
(± SEM)	(0.021)	(0.045)	(0.027)	(0.036)	(0.023)	(0.025)	(0.049)
Aphasic patients	−0.013	−0.033	−0.009	0.019	−0.046***	−0.032	−0.212*
(± SEM)	(0.095)	(0.106)	(0.091)	(0.041)	(0.054)	(0.077)	(0.110)
Nonaphasic patients	0.161	0.096	0.177	0.146	0.142	0.011	0.081
(± SEM)	(0.094)	(0.203)	(0.106)	(0.052	(0.064)	(0.045	(0.087)
Verbal/foreign language index							
Normals	0.068	0.044	0.012	0.102	0.110	0.058	0.062
(± SEM)	(0.026)	(0.079)	(0.040)	(0.024)	(0.037)	(0.028)	(0.039)
Aphasic patients	0.012	0.114	0.042	0.018	−0.027	−0.084	−0.296**
(± SEM)	(0.199)	(0.153)	(0.143)	(0.082)	(0.060)	(0.094)	(0.130)
Nonaphasic patients	0.039	−0.149	−0.004	0.107	0.027	0.032	0.044
(± SEM)	(0.036)	(0.139)	(0.068)	(0.048)	(0.046)	(0.077)	(0.131)

* $p < 0.05$; ** $p < 0.01$; *** $p < 0.005$.

Results

Patients with Ischemic Cerebrovascular Disease

The index of ratios on total power and power associated with single frequency bands for verbal/musical, verbal/white noise, verbal/foreign language tasks are presented in table I. The verbal/musical index for total power was lower, but not significant, in aphasic patients compared to the normal subjects and the nonaphasic brain-lesioned patients. There were no significant differences in the index for the delta, theta-1 and theta-2 bands between the aphasic patients and the other 2 groups, but it was significantly lower for the alpha (t-test; $p < 0.005$) and beta-2 bands ($p < 0.05$) in the aphasics.

The evident decrease for the alpha band index in aphasic subjects during verbal/musical tasks, observed in mean values, did not occur in all cases: 4 patients showed similar and sometimes higher values compared to those found in normal subjects (fig. 1). The particular trend found in the 4 patients cannot be explained by a different degree of aphasia, as the aphasia was very severe. In all the patients with scores ranging between 0 and 8 there were no substantial differences between cases with low index values and the 4 patients with high values (fig. 2). Three patients with low values were analyzed again about a month later, when they showed a clear improvement in the language impairment. In two of them the index had increased to within the range observed in normal subjects.

The group of nonaphasic brain-lesioned patients, in which mean values were not significantly different from those of normals, also included 4 patients with lower values in the verbal/musical index compared to the normal subjects.

The verbal/foreign language index values below zero involved only the alpha and beta frequencies in the aphasic patients, but with the exception of the beta-2 band ($p < 0.01$) the differences were not significant. In the nonaphasic patients, the delta and theta-1 bands gave values below zero, but there were no significant differences in any band compared to the normal subjects.

Epileptic Patients

During verbal/musical tasks, the patients with temporal lobe epilepsy showed mean values of the index significantly lower than those of normals for the alpha band ($p < 0.001$) and for the beta-1 band ($p < 0.05$) (fig. 3).

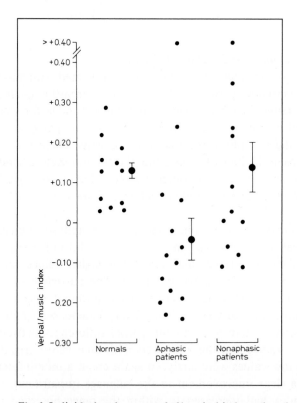

Fig. 1. Individual and mean verbal/musical index values (± SEM) for alpha power.

The index of the verbal/foreign language produced a significant decrease for the alpha and beta-1 bands ($p < 0.01$).

In order to exclude the possibility that interindividual differences could be linked to a different level of vigilance induced by antiepileptic drugs, simple reaction times were assessed. Mean values in the epileptics were 290 ± 80.2 ms, ranging from 217 to 439, slower than those found in age-matched normal subjects in our laboratory. However, this different degree of delay in reaction times among individual patients was not correlated with the different alpha band index values observed during verbal/musical tasks. Likewise, a comparison of this index for the alpha band with serum phenobarbital, carbamazepine and phenytoin levels, taking into account the fact that 30% of patients were on polytherapy, revealed no relation between the 2 parameters.

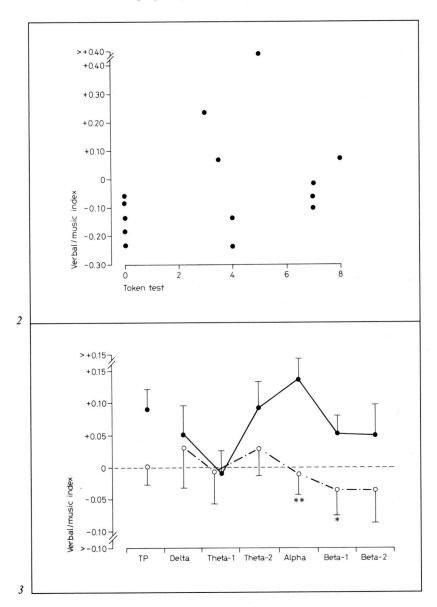

Fig. 2. Individual verbal/musical index values for alpha power in aphasic patients in relation to aphasia severity.

Fig. 3. Mean verbal/musical index values for total power (TP) and power associated with single frequency bands in normals (full circles) and in epileptic patients (empty circles); t-test: * p < 0.05; ** p < 0.001.

Discussion

The technique described, applied to the analysis of the EEG recording from parieto-occipital regions, has proved to be a suitable means of detecting the presence of language disorders in brain-lesioned patients. The parieto-occipital site was preferred to others on the basis of our experience with normal subjects, in whom these bipolar derivations were particularly effective in revealing variations depending on different types of auditory tasks [44], and because recordings from these regions seem to provide data which can be better correlated with regional cerebral blood flow variations in patients with vascular brain diseases [50, 54].

In patients with right hemiplegia following supratentorial unilateral infarction, there was a homolateral depression in the alpha rhythm, already described by Berger in 2 cases [31], and a remarkable quantity of slow waves particularly on the left. This slow activity, which reflects a metabolic depression or a reduction in blood flow [30, 32, 45], was prevalent in patients with language disorders, but differences were not sufficient to distinguish these patients from those without language disorders.

Analysis based on task-dependent EEG asymmetry, on the other hand, does allow a distinction among patients according to the presence or absence of language comprehension deficits, determined mainly through verbal and musical tasks. This could indicate that the verbal stimulus has lost its cognitive connotation for aphasic patients, while their capacity to analyze music, considered to belong mainly to the right hemisphere [see ref. 18], remains unimpaired. This hypothesis would explain clinical observations that these patients maintain the melody of language, and that musicians with aphasia can continue in their work [3], and also justify the use of melodic intonation in language therapy [52].

It would therefore seem that low verbal/musical task index values do not depend solely on a lesser involvement of the left side during the verbal task but that there is also an active right-side prevalence during the musical task. If the low values of this index were due only to a lesser left-side activity during the verbal task, the same trend would have emerged with the verbal/foreign language index, while the values given by this index did not differ significantly from those of normal subjects.

Haaland and Wertz [28], studying 10 aphasic patients, of whom 4 were classified as severe and 6 as mild to moderate, did not find clear modifications in interhemispheric asymmetry in relation to the tasks (word-picture), but they did observe less left-hemispheric activity in the

severe aphasic patients. We did not find a relation between index values
and the severity of the aphasia, but in 2 patients who showed a normaliza-
tion of language impairment over a period of about one month, the trend
observed during verbal/musical tasks became similar to that found in normal subjects.

This technique also appears appropriate, if less obviously, for the
detection of verbal cognitive function variations in temporal lobe epileptic
patients with left EEG focus and without clinically detectable language
disorders. Considered as a group, these epileptics presented verbal/musical
index values significantly lower than those of the control subjects during
verbal and musical tasks, confirming the results obtained by our group [26,
43] and by others [2]. There were, however, interindividual variations
which were not related to different serum levels of the antiepileptic drugs
nor to the extent of delays in simple reaction times. The frequently low
index would thus appear to be independent of the level of vigilance and
also of the extent of the cerebral lesion since patients with normal CT scan
were considered.

These electrophysiological data, indicating that epileptics with left
temporal EEG focus have some difficulty in processing verbal tasks, are in
agreement with the greater frequency of verbal disorders in these patients
[12, 25, 34, 38]. The metabolic depression on the site of EEG interictal
focus, observed directly with PET [11, 35] or indirectly with SPECT [4], is
broader than the EEG abnormalities. This great metabolic impairment
could justify alterations in verbal cognitive elaboration in these patients
and thus explain our abnormal electrophysiological findings. Task-dependent EEG asymmetry thus appears as a functional exploration technique
capable of revealing cognitive function disorders in brain-lesioned patients.

References

1   Adrian, E.; Matthews, B.: The Berger rhythm: potential changes from the occipital
    lobes in man. Brain 57: 355–385 (1934).
2   Angeleri, F.; Signorino, O.; Provinciali, L.: Hemispheric specialization in general-
    ized and partial epilepsy: a study of cerebral asymmetry in P300 and alpha waves
    during selected acoustic stimulations. Res. Commun. Psychol. Psychiat. Behav. 12:
    33–51 (1987).
3   Assal, G.: Aphasie de Wernicke sans amusie chez un pianiste. Revue neurol. 129:
    251–255 (1973).
4   Biersack, H.; Reichmann, K.: Winkler, C.; Stefan, H.; Kuhen, K.; Bulau, P.; Penin,

H.; Tyrrel, D.; Neirinkx, R.; Grumer, K.: 99m Tc-labelled hexamethylpropyleneamineoxime photon emission scans in epilepsy. Lancet *ii:* 1436–1437 (1985).

5   Blinkov, S.; Moskatova, A.: Paradoxical decrease of the reaction time in focal epilepsy. Cortex *12:* 219–232 (1976).

6   Bogen, J.E.; Gordon, H.: Musical tests for functional lateralization with intracarotid amobarbital. Nature *230:* 524–525 (1971).

7   Butler, S.; Glass, A.: EEG correlates of cerebral dominance, in Riesen, Thompson, Advances in psychobiology, vol. 3, pp. 219–272 (Wiley, New York 1976).

8   Cornil, L.; Gastaut, H.: Etude électroencéphalographique de la dominance sensorielle d'un hémisphère cérébral. Presse méd. *37:* 421–422 (1947).

9   De Renzi, E.; Faglioni, P.: Normative data and screening power of a shortened version of the Token test. Cortex *14:* 41–49 (1978).

10   Donchin, E.; Kutas, M.; McCarty, G.: Electrocortical indices of hemispheric utilization; in Harnard, Doty, Goldstein, Jaynes, Krauthamer, Lateralization in the nervous system, pp. 339–384 (Academic Press, New York 1977).

11   Engel, J.; Kuhl, D.; Phelps, M.; Crandall, P.: Comparative localization of epileptic foci in partial epilepsy by PCT and EEG. Ann. Neurol. *12:* 529–537 (1982).

12   Fedio, P.; Mirsky, A.: Selective intellectual deficits in children with temporal lobe or centroencephalic epilepsy. Neuropsychology *7:* 267–300 (1969).

13   Furst, J.: EEG alpha asymmetry and visuospatial performance. Nature *260:* 254–255 (1976).

14   Galin, D.; Ornstein, R.; Kocel, K.; Merrin, E.: Hemispheric localization of cognitive mode by EEG. Psychophysiology *8:* 246–247 (1971).

15   Galin, D.; Ornstein, R.: Lateral specialization of cognitive mode: an EEG study. Psychophysiology *9:* 412–418 (1972).

16   Galin, D.; Johnstone, J.; Herron, J.: Effects of task difficulty on EEG measures of cerebral engagement. Neuropsychology *16:* 461–472 (1978).

17   Galin, D.; Ornstein, R.; Herron, J.; Johnstone, J.: Sex and handedness differences in EEG measures of hemispheric specialization. Brain Lang. *16:* 19–55 (1982).

18   Gates, A.; Bradshaw, J.: The role of the cerebral hemispheres in music. Brain Lang. *4:* 403–431 (1977).

19   Gevins, D.; Zeitlin, G.; Yingling, C.; Doyle, J.; Dedon, M.; Schaffer, R.; Ruomasset, J.; Yager, C.: EEG patterns during 'cognitive' tasks. I. Methodology and analysis of complex behaviours. Electroenceph. clin. Neurophysiol. *47:* 693–703 (1979).

20   Gevins, D.; Zeitlin, G.; Doyle, J.; Schaffer, R.; Callaway, E.: EEG patterns during 'cognitive' tasks. II. Analysis of controlled tasks. Electroenceph. clin. Neurophysiol. *47:* 704–710 (1979).

21   Giannitrapani, D.; Sorkin, A.; Ernenstein, J.: Laterality preference of children and adults as related to interhemispheric EEG phase activity. J. neurol. Sci. *3:* 139–150 (1966).

22   Giannitrapani, D.: Localization of language and arithmetic functions via EEG factor analysis. Res. Commun. Psychol. Psychiat. Behav. *7:* 39–55 (1982).

23   Glanville, A.; Antonitis, J.: The relationship between occipital alpha activity and laterality. J. exp. Psychol. *49:* 295–299 (1955).

24   Glass, A.; Butler, S.: Alpha EEG asymmetry and speed of left hemisphere thinking. Neurosci. Lett. *4:* 231–235 (1977).

25 Glowinsky, H.: Cognitive deficits in temporal lobe epilepsy. J. nerv. ment. Dis. *157:* 129–137 (1973).
26 Goldstein, L.; Denoth, F.; Murri, L.; Stefanini, A.; Muratorio, A.: Automatic computerized analysis of hemispheric EEG relationships in neurotic and epileptic patients; in Perris, van Knorring, Clinical neurophysiological aspects of psychopathological conditions, pp. 3–13 (Karger, Basel 1980).
27 Goldstein, L.: Some EEG correlates of behavioral traits states in human. Res. Commun. Psychol. Psychiat. Behav. *8:* 115–141 (1983).
28 Haaland, K.; Wertz, R.: Interhemispheric EEG activity in normal and aphasic adults. Percept. Mot. Skills *42:* 827–833 (1976).
29 Hirshkowitz, M.; Earle, J.; Paley, B.: EEG alpha asymmetry in musicians and non musicians. A study of hemispheric specialization. Neuropsychology *16:* 125–128 (1978).
30 Ingvar, D.: The pathophysiology of occlusive cerebrovascular disorders related to neuroradiological findings, EEG and measurements of regional cerebral blood flow. Acta neurol. scand. *43:* suppl. 31, pp. 93–107 (1967).
31 Jasper, H.: Electrical signs of cortical activity. Psychol. Bull. *34:* 411–481 (1937).
32 Jonkman, E.: Cerebral blood flow (CBF) and electrical activity (EEG); in Minderhoud, Cerebral blood flow: basic knowledge and clinical implications, pp. 202–222 (Excerpta Medica, Amsterdam 1981).
33 Kimura, D.: Left-right differences in the perception of melodies. Q.Jl Psychol. *6:* 335–358 (1964).
34 Ladavas, E.; Umiltá, C.; Provinciali, L.: Hemisphere dependent cognitive performances in epileptic patients. Epilepsia *20:* 493–502 (1979).
35 Latack, J.; Abou-Khalil, B.; Siegel, J.; Sackellares, J.; Gabrielsen, T.; Aisen, A.: Patients with partial seizures: evaluation by MR, CT, and PET imaging. Radiology *159:* 159–163 (1986).
36 Leissner, P.; Lindholm, L.; Petersen, I.: Alpha amplitude dependence on skull thickness as measured by ultrasound technique. Electroenceph. clin. Neurophysiol. *29:* 392–399 (1970).
37 Le May, M.; Geschwind, N.: Asymmetries of the human cerebral hemispheres; in Caramazza, Zurif, Language acquisition and language breakdown: paralleles and divergences, pp. 311–328 (Johns Hopkins University Press, Baltimore 1978).
38 Mayeux, R.; Brandt, J.; Rosen, J.; Benson, D.: Interictal memory and language impairment in temporal lobe epilepsy. Neurology *30:* 120–125 (1980).
39 Mazzucchi, A.; Parma, M.: Responses to dichotic listening tasks in temporal epileptics with or without clinically evident lesions. Cortex *14:* 381–390 (1978).
40 McKee, G.; Humphery, B.; McAdam, D.W.: Scaled lateralization of alpha activity during linguistic and musical tasks. Psychophysiology *10:* 441–443 (1973).
41 Milner, B.: Psychological aspects of focal epilepsy and its neurosurgical management; in Purpura, Penry, Walter, Neurosurgical management of the epilepsies. Adv. Neurol., vol. 8, pp. 299–321 (Raven Press, New York 1975).
42 Morgan, A.H.; MacDonald, P.J.; MacDonald, H.: Differences in bilateral alpha activity as a function of experimental task with a note on lateral eye movements and hypnotizability. Neuropsychology *9:* 459–469 (1971).

43 Murri, L.; Stefanini, A.; Bonanni, E.; Muratorio, A.; Goldstein, L.; Navona, C.; Denoth, F.: Analisi automatica dell'asimmetria interemisferica EEG nelle sindromi epilettiche. Boll. Lega It. Epil. *45:* 199–203 (1984).
44 Murri, L.; Muratorio, A.; Stefanini, A.; Navona, C.; Denoth, F.: Asimmetria EEG e specializzazione emisferica. Riv. It. EEG Neurofisiol. Clin., suppl. 1, pp. 241–265 (1984).
45 Nagata, K.; Tagawa, K.; Shishido, F.; Uemura, K.: Topographic EEG correlates of cerebral blood flow and oxygen consumption in patients with neuropsychological disorders; in Duffy, Topographic mapping of brain electrical activity, pp. 357–370 (Butterworth, Boston 1984).
46 Oldfield, R.: The assessment of analysis of handedness: The Edinburgh inventory. Neuropsychology *9:* 93–113 (1971).
47 Ornestein, R.; Johnstone, J.; Swencionis, C.; Herron, J.: Differential right hemisphere engagement in visuospatial tasks. Neuropsychology *18:* 49–64 (1980).
48 Provins, K.; Cunliffe, P.: The relationship between EEG activity and handedness. Cortex *8:* 136–146 (1972).
49 Raney, E.: Brain potentials and lateral dominance in identical twins. J. exp. Psychol. *24:* 21–39 (1939).
50 Samson-Dollfus, D.; Rogier, M.; Souliac, B.: Application de l'analyse spectrale de l'EEG à l'étude de malades atteints d'insuffisance vasculaire cérébrale. Rev. Electroencéphalogr. Neurophysiol. clin. *6:* 328–329 (1976).
51 Shepherd, R.; Gale, A.: EEG correlates of hemisphere differences during a rapid calculation task. Br. J. Psychol. *73:* 73–84 (1982).
52 Sparks, R.; Helm, N.; Albert, M.: Aphasia rehabilitation resulting from melodic intonation therapy. Cortex *10:* 303–316 (1974).
53 Sperry, R.: Lateral specialization in the surgically separated hemispheres; in Schmitt, Worden, The neurosciences. Third Study Program (MIT Press, Cambridge 1974).
54 Tolonen, U.; Sulg, I.A.: Comparison of quantitative EEG parameters from four different analysis techniques in evaluation of relationship between EEG and CBF in brain infarction. Electroenceph. clin. Neurophysiol. *1:* 177–185 (1981).
55 Wada, J.; Clarke, R.; Hamm, A.: Cerebral hemispheric asymmetry in humans. Archs Neurol. *32:* 239–246 (1975).
56 Wogan, M.; Moore, S.; Epro, R.; Harner, R.: EEG measures of alternative strategies used by subjects to solve block designs. Int. J. Neurosci. *12:* 25–28 (1981).

Luigi Murri, MD, Servizio di Neurofisiopatologia, Clinica Neurologica, Università di Pisa, Via Roma 67, I-56100 Pisa (Italy)

Giannitrapani, Murri (eds.), The EEG of Mental Activities,
pp. 119–135 (Karger, Basel 1988)

Hemispheric Specialization in Normal, Cerebrovascular and Epileptic Subjects

A Study by EEG Power Spectra and Evoked Potentials during Neuropsychological Test

Franco Angeleri, Mario Signorino, Leandro Provinciali, Osvaldo Scarpino

Istituto Policattedra delle Malattie del Sistema Nervoso, Università di Ancona, Ancona, Italy

A large amount of anatomical, clinical and experimental data [16] suggests an asymmetrical engagement of selected cortical areas during specific performances. This condition is generally known as 'hemispheric specialization'. At the present time the basis and limits of this concept are not well defined, mainly because its underlying neural mechanisms are as yet poorly understood.

Though neurophysiology has been late in approaching this topic [8], one of its branches, electrophysiology, may be considered a valid mean of studying it. Currently, the hypotheses proposed to explain the different hemispheric functions agree that the anatomo-functional basis of hemispheric specialization is based upon the cortical neuronal activity where the bioelectrical brain potentials are generated [11, 15, 25, 30, 39, 48, 52, 53]. Both nonstationary (time domain; evoked potentials = EP) and stationary (frequency domain; EEG power spectra) electrical potentials may be studied using electrophysiological techniques to investigate possible correlations between a functional engagement of one hemisphere and bioelectrical phenomena of either short or long duration. The most recent contributions to this research seem to demonstrate that electrophysiological methods are a valid approach to improve our knowledge of hemispheric specialization. Further information may be found in Giannitrapani's recent monograph [33]. In a review of the topic and original investigations, the author reaches interesting and stimulating conclusions, of

which the following must be quoted in particular. Some frequency components of steady-state EEG correlate with higher cortical functions; the cortical location of these functions can be detected using an EEG factorial
analysis; such methods have confirmed the left lateralization of Broca's
area and have also shown that the right temporal areas play an important
role in the search for perceptual organization.

The aim of the present paper is to summarize and discuss the results of
our research in this field, but first of all, it is useful to examine some
information emerging from the literature about the investigations which
have employed EEG methods based upon either the frequency or time
domain analysis.

EEG Analysis in the Frequency Domain

A simple visual inspection of EEG tracings shows changes related to
various functional conditions of the brain, e.g. wakefulness or sleep, psy-
chosensorial rest or mental concentration [41]. Therefore, if physiological
EEG changes reveal different functional conditions of the brain, it may be
hypothesized that lateralized or localized functions may also be expressed
by diffuse or focal variations in the brain's bioelectrical potentials. However, a simple visual inspection of an EEG tracing is not enough to distinguish EEG changes related to the engagement of localized neuronal pools,
such as those assumed to be responsible for specific functions. Some
authors have suggested more sophisticated methods of EEG signal analysis
with the aim of overcoming the limits of visual EEG inspection [see the
review by Donchin et al., 18].

Giannitrapani [26] introduced the log amplitude score and the phase
angle score of EEG bands; Giannitrapani [27] and Galin and Ornstein [22]
employed the conventional EEG spectral analysis. Morgan et al. [44] proposed a filtered EEG analysis, Butler and Glass [12] the compilation of
amplitude histograms, Chartok et al. [14] the measurement of the variation
in the alpha bands with time, Callaway and Harris [13] and Yingling [55]
the detection of the cortical coupling index.

Wide disagreement exists about the best method of detecting the
hemispheric EEG activity when a lateralized task is performed. The spectral analysis of the EEG is the method most widely used processing stationary potentials [29]. The log ratio of the left and right EEG band amplitude
derived from homologous bihemispheric sites is considered an index of the

hemispheric engagement. Amplitude reduction of the EEG signal in the explored area is considered as corresponding to the cortical engagement for a specific function in that area. Thus, ratio values greater than 1 mean an engagement of the left hemisphere, less than 1 an engagement of the right. However, this figure must not be considered an absolute measure of the degree of the hemispheric engagement. The EEG band amplitude ratio also depends on the basal condition in which the two hemispheres are working. In other words, the shift of the left/right ratio must be considered as evidence of the engagement of the former or the latter hemisphere regardless of the absolute value of the ratio [24].

Furthermore, it must be stressed that many conditions influence the detectable degree of asymmetry in the EEG activity. Regardless of the electrical flow changes depending on specific engagement of neuronal aggregates, the following factors must be mentioned: the thickness of the skull (filtering effect of the skull), the possible existence of lesions without clinical symptomatology underneath the recording electrodes and, finally, the 'mentation' of the subject during the tasks. As well as the quoted difficulties related to intra and inter subject differences, the positioning of active electrodes and the reference electrode may be a source of errors in the interpretation of the results [50]. In conclusion it must be underlined that the validity of the final results is strictly linked to the use of correct techniques and a suitable choice of methods.

Most investigations into electrical asymmetries of the hemispheres due to the execution of selective tasks have been based upon the following experimental conditions: (1) active and checked performance of a task presumed to be activating one hemisphere only; (2) 'mentation' situations imposed by the test procedure or induced by prolonged stimulations and presumed to be activating one hemisphere only; (3) comparison between subjects functionally considered as 'left or right hemispherically engaged' because of their professional activity or cognitive style; (4) subject performance and EEG recording during different states of consciousness induced by hypnosis, biofeedback or sleep, during which different spontaneous engagement of the hemispheres is presumed. As far as the last item is concerned the studies are motivated by the hypothesis that dream activity derives from a right hemisphere engagement because of its visuospatial and holistic characteristics [3, 34, 45].

From the many investigations carried out using the above-mentioned methods the following conclusions may be drawn [7, 17, 18, 32]. It is possible to engage one hemisphere only by appropriate tasks and/or stimulations based upon the quoted experimental criteria. Either a total or selective reduction in the amplitude of the EEG power spectra bands is observed during the performance of such tests.

EEG Analysis in the Time Domain (Evoked Potentials)

The EP can be divided into three groups of components: (1) early components: expression of the synaptic activation of the subcortical pathways (far field components) and of the primary sensory cortex; (2) middle range components: expression of the activation of the primary and secondary sensory cortex; (3) late components: expression of the activation of the secondary and associative sensory cortex.

Middle and late components may be elicited and/or influenced by the kind of stimuli and experimental conditions. Among the late components, the P300 wave is thought to be strictly related to cognitive information processing and it has also been defined as an 'endogenous' EP or event-related potential, because of its underlying mechanisms. The CNV is similarly related to attentive and cognitive processes, and therefore it can be included among the event-related potentials.

Investigations carried out using EP methods are able to demonstrate the existence of a hemispheric specialization, and to identify the steps through which a given lateralized process takes place. Language studies offer examples of this. The word which acts as the key to understanding the meaning of the sentence may be clearly identified by EP methods (greater P300 amplitude at the keyword); similarly the mutual relations within a linguistic structure can be detected (greater P300 amplitude in relation to the estimated stimulus expectancy).

Criticisms of the electrophysiological methods have been advanced [18, 20]. Nevertheless, authors generally agree that EP methods can detect different lateralized areas of the two hemispheres if procedural rules are respected and experimental conditions are based upon a specific lateralized engagement (i.e. active and controlled performance of a verbal or spatial task, subject's mentation about a verbal or spatial matter). Furthermore, Wood [54], using the EP method, has confirmed the difference existing between auditory and phonetic 'processing' of an acoustic verbal stimulus, the former being able to analyze the nonverbal features of the stimulus, the latter being able to process the stimulus so as to extract its abstract phonetic features.

The experimental set-ups involving the use of EP have problems analogous to those using the ongoing EEG spectral analysis. In particular, since the period analyzed by means of the EP is very short, the 'mentation' and the different strategies chosen by the subjects during the task assume particular importance when cognitive processes are studied. In order to overcome this limitation, the subject is required to use only one of the various cognitive options available; furthermore, a confirmation of the cognitive process chosen by the subject is sought.

Besides the accuracy of the experimental set and the statistical analysis of the results [20, 37], the interpretation of the computerized signals causes other difficulties. EP amplitude and latency variations may involve the whole potential or some of their components. The amplitude asymmetry of the whole potential may reflect the hemispheric specialization, defined as (1) the different size of neural pool that generate the EP [23, 47], or (2) the result of the most direct access of the input to a hemisphere [11].

Some authors suggest that information processing is only partially lateralized and such lateralization is reflected by the amplitude asymmetry of some EP components yet some criticism of this interpretation has been reported [40].

Similarly the EP latency asymmetries may be due to the most direct access to one hemisphere [11] or to chronological differences between the two hemispheres in processing the information. The latter condition would apply particularly to the 'endogenous' EP components.

Finally, some particular features of the stimulus selectively activating one hemisphere must be stressed: for example, the importance of exposure duration, luminance, stimulus size, spatial frequency, luminance contrast, and retinal eccentricity is well known when a visual stimulus is employed. All these elements shift the prevalence of stimulus processing from one hemisphere to the other or they cancel the prevalent function of the former, affecting both the EP amplitude and latency at the same time.

Personal Contribution

EEG Power Spectra and EP in Normal Subjects during
Wakefulness and Sleep
The holistic and visuospatial characteristics of dreams support the hypothesis that a functional hemispheric asymmetry with greater right activation can exist during REM sleep. Experimental evidence strengthen-

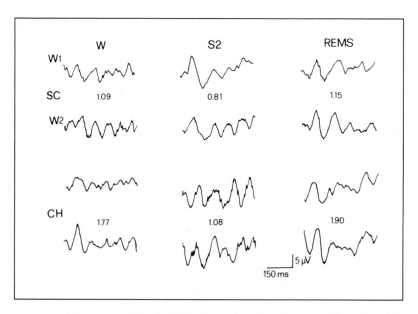

Fig. 1. Evoked responses from the left (W1) and the right (W2) side of the scalp of one subject to the presentation of stop consonant (SC) and chords (CH) during wakefulness (W), stage 2 (S2) and REM sleep (REMS). Numbers between responses represent the values of the right/left N1–P2 amplitude ratio. From ref. [3]; the study was carried out on 6 subjects.

ing this assumption was obtained using a different approach. Angeleri et al. [3] studied the correlation between neurophysiological and neuropsychological data obtained under the same experimental conditions in 6 healthy male right-handed subjects. Both musical stimuli (chords) and verbal stimuli (stop consonants) were used to elicit the EP, which were recorded from the temporo-parietal areas. Electrodes were fixed by collodion at the center of a triangle made by location P3, T3 and T5 of the 10–20 system, close to Wernicke's area (W1) and at the homologous opposite are (W2) according to Matsumiya et al. [43]. Linked mastoid electrodes were used as reference. The EEG power spectra were recorded while the subject was listening to a musical selection (musical stimulus) and a verbal passage (verbal stimulus). Each stimulus was administered twice in sleep (S2 and REM stages) and once in wakefulness (W).

The electrophysiological data were correlated with both the awakening effect induced by the stimulation and with the mental activity preceding

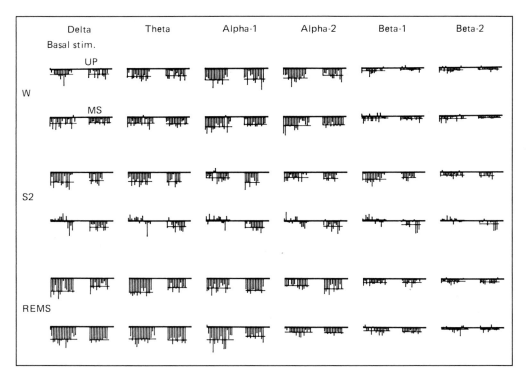

Fig. 2. Right/left power ratios of a subject for each frequency band, physiological state (wakefulness = W, stage 2 sleep = S2, REM sleep = REMS) and experimental condition (basal and stimulus conditions, verbal passage = VP, musical selection = MS). Horizontal thick lines represent abscissae; vertical lines are logarithmic values of right/left power ratios with the mean value for each period drawn as a horizontal thin line. From ref. [3]; the study was carried out on 6 subjects.

the stimulation. They were analyzed with respect to the subject's report, according to the criteria suggested by Foulkes and Pope [19].

Two peaks prevailed as the most stable and constant EP components, i.e. N1 and P2, with a mean latency of 108 and 185 ms, respectively. Regardless of the stimulus condition, there was a decrease in the right/left amplitude ratio of the responses obtained by stimulation during wakefulness and in S2, whereas there was an increase in this ratio during REM stimulation (fig. 1).

Figure 2 shows power spectrum changes due to physiological states and stimulus characteristics. Significant changes in the right/left power ratio occurred in the delta and theta bands during the 'musical' condition in stage 2 and during the 'verbal' condition in the REM stage.

The results confirm the existence of a functional hemispheric asymmetry during sleep, that is, the right hemisphere predominating during the REM stage. It is confirmed that different physiological conditions determine an asymmetric activation but the subject's specific mental content seems to be a more important factor.

EP in Normal Subjects during Visual Half-Field Stimulation Using a Grating Pattern

Several authors [49] suggest that hemispheric specialization already takes place at the earliest level of stimulus processing, that is, at the sensory level. It is similarly accepted that the early and middle-range EP components reflect primary sensory cortex engagement. Therefore it may be hypothesized that there is a different topographical distribution in both the latency and amplitude of the cortical EP component, when employing a grating, whose neural processing is assumed to be lateralized.

In order to assess this hypothesis, Signorino et al. [51] have recorded visual EP using a method of visual half-field stimulation in 5 healthy right-handed subjects, the stimulus adopted being a vertical grating pattern reversal whose spatial frequency composition can be considered simpler than the checkerboard. Under these stimulus conditions, the EP are characterized by 3 peaks, labelled N1, P1, N2, the greatest amplitude being that of the N1–P1 complex monitored in the right occipital areas, independent of the half-field stimulated (table I). Barrett et al. [6] have observed that

Table I. Visual EP components in the right-, mid- and left-occipital areas under right and left half-field stimulation

	Right half-field			Left half-field		
	RO	MO	LO	RO	MO	LO
Lat N1, ms	72.5 ± 6.2	72.4 ± 5.0	72.5 ± 12.2	70.5 ± 21.2	71.3 ± 11.6	73.5 ± 7.5
Lat P1, ms	102.5 ± 7.5	105.5 ± 10.8	105.5 ± 18.7	102.6 ± 17.5	103.7 ± 6.4	105.0 ± 6.2
Lat N2, ms	151.0 ± 27.5	161.0 ± 33.3	154.5 ± 31.2	150.0 ± 27.5	154.7 ± 22.4	152.8 ± 9.8
Amp N1–P1, µV	4.9 ± 1.7	3.8 ± 1.9	1.7 ± 0.4	3.6 ± 1.9	3.1 ± 2.4	$3.1 \pm 0.8*$
Amp P1–N2, µV	4.7 ± 1.4	4.5 ± 3.0	3.2 ± 1.2	4.7 ± 8	3.0 ± 1.6	3.3 ± 0.8

* $p < 0.05$.

the amplitude of the checkerboard pattern EP is greater in the occipital area ipsilateral to the half-field stimulated, thus suggesting that such a paradoxical phenomenon depends on the orientation of the excitation dipole with respect to the recording electrodes.

This phenomenon was not observed in the experiments performed by Signorino et al. [51]. In fact, this study differs from Barrett et al. [6] in that the use of a simpler pattern and binocular vision activates direct and crossed afferent fibers, so modifying the orientation of the excitation dipole.

Moreover, since no execution of a cognitive task was required during visual stimulation in the experiment performed by Signorino et al. [51], the greater amplitude of the N1–P1 complexes in the right occipital areas must be interpreted as a phenomenon which expresses the lateralized processing of the stimulus at sensory level. In addition, it must be remembered that the black-and-white square-wave vertical grating used stimulus was of spatial frequency equal to 1c/deg with 80% contrast. It was displayed on a TV screen at a distance of 140 cm from the subject's nasion, presented to both right and left visual half-fields, and viewed binocularly. EP were recorded from 3 electrodes, one placed on the midline 5 cm above the inion (MO), and the others on the right (RO) and left (LO) 5 cm lateral to the MO. All electrodes were referred to a common frontal electrode placed 12 cm above the nasion over the midline.

EEG Power Spectra and EP Recorded during Single and
Simultaneous Intermittent Verbal Task:
A Study in Normal Subjects and Patients Affected by Mild Brain Atrophy
Rhodes et al. [46], Bigum et al. [9], Galbraith et al. [21], Grunau et al. [38] studied the differences between the two hemispheres in patients affected by a global impairment of language or memory, while Giannitrapani and Kayton [28], Goldstein and Harnad [35], Giannitrapani [31] and Liberson and Fried [42] investigated the same differences in patients with psychic disorders.

These studies demonstrate that methods based upon EEG spectral power analysis allows an evaluation of the disorder of some cognitive functions associated to either discrete cerebral lesions or alterations without anatomical damage. Furthermore, if a cognitive function is altered, not abolished, the resulting neuropsychological changes and their electrophysiological correlates offer some clue to the neural mechanisms which underlie the same function.

From this starting point Angeleri et al. [2] studied two groups of subjects in order to evaluate interhemispheric EEG asymmetries when the brain's verbal areas are active. The first group consisted of 5 normal, young subjects, and the second was a group of 5 60-year-old men with a diffuse cerebral atrophy but without clinical evidence of language defects. All subjects performed two different verbal tasks.

During the first task the subjects had to recognize whether a visual presentation of four stop consonants was the same as or different from another sequence administered 5 s before through earphones (standard task). In the second task this was repeated while the subject was counting backwards in threes (task with interference).

The CNV and P300 were obtained by averaging selected EEG tracings starting from 0.5 s before acoustic stimulation and finishing 1 s after visual stimulation. Electrodes were fixed at the center of a triangle made by location P3, T3 and T5 of the 10–20 system, close to Wernicke's area (W1) and at the homologous area (W2). Linked-mastoid electrodes were used as reference.

The same experiment was used to detect the different effect of verbal stimuli on the background EEG activity of the two hemispheres. With this aim, EEG tracings monitored from right and left parieto-temporal areas were analyzed in the 4-second epochs between the acoustic and visual presentation.

The EP results showed a well-defined CNV recurring under both experimental conditions in all subjects: its amplitude, however, was greater in the group of young subjects and during the task without interference. No significant asymmetry in the CNV amplitude was ever observed. The mean P300 latency was 345 ± 14 ms in the first group of subjects, and 398 ± 32 in the second group. The longest latencies in both groups occurred in the task with interference. The second group showed a significantly lower P300 amplitude. No interhemispheric asymmetry in P300 latency and amplitude was observed in both groups.

There was a constant asymmetry in the spectral power of the alpha band during the first task (standard task without interference) in both groups examined (normal control and subjects with cerebral atrophy). During the second task the asymmetry decreased in normal subjects; conversely, in subjects with cerebral atrophy, the interhemispheric asymmetry increased due to an increase in alpha power in the right hemisphere.

The data obtained confirm the alpha band asymmetry of EEG power spectra during verbal tasks. Its increased difficulty, due to verbal interference, modifies the interhemispheric asymmetry of the alpha band. Different features occur between normal and aged subjects. The former group showed an increase of EEG alpha power from the left parieto-temporal area (W1); likewise, subjects included in this group obtained good scores in the tasks. On the contrary in the latter group the alpha power increase was greater in the right parieto-temporal area (W2), such a condition corresponding to a decrease of neuropsychological performance. On the basis of these results a correlation between verbal performance and EEG findings may be proposed; they also demonstrate a different hemispheric involvement in normal and abnormal subjects.

On the contrary EP obtained from the same cortical areas (W1, W2) showed no interhemispheric difference of latency and amplitude in both groups, but a longer latency of EP was documented in older subjects (second group). The last finding confirms previous investigations [1, 36] which indicates that EP are a suitable method to detect slight brain damage.

EEG Power Spectra and EP during Lateralized Stimuli in Epileptic Patients

Because of localized or diffuse changes of EEG activity which occur in epileptic syndromes whether primitive or secondary, partial or generalized, it may be supposed that epilepsy is a good natural model for investigating hemispheric specialization. Much neuropsychological evidence exists on the disturbance of cognitive functions in epileptics; through the lateralization of an epileptic focus, even if nonlesional, it is possible to establish changes in cognitive lateralized functions.

It may also be supposed that the model of human epilepsy is useful for investigating whether the electrophysiological correlates of hemispheric specialization persist in the presence of altered neuronal excitability.

On the basis of these considerations, Angeleri et al. [4, 5] have investigated the possible existence of functional hemispheric asymmetry during tasks involving lateralized processing performed by 15 epileptics (5 generalized nonconvulsive, 10 partial, of whom 5 had a left and 5 had a right non-lesional focus) and in 5 normal subjects. The hemispheric asymmetry was evaluated by processing the log ratio of right/left R/L EEG power spectra and EP amplitude and using musical and verbal stimuli to elicit a differentiated right or left hemisphere engagement. The recording electrodes were fixed at the center of a triangle made by location T3 and T5 of the 10–20 system, close to the Wernicke's area (W1) and at the homologous opposite area (W2). Linked-mastoid electrodes were used as reference.

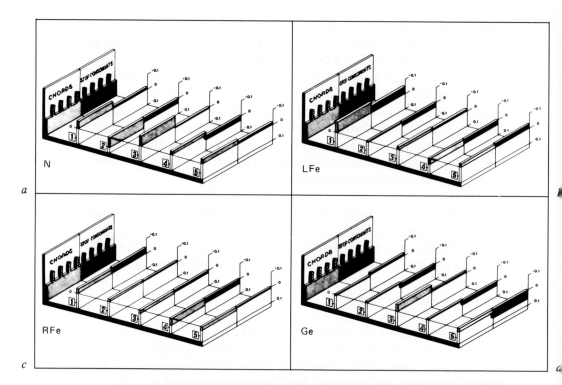

Fig. 3. Log R/L values of the P300 amplitude during stimulation with chords and stop consonants. *a–d* All subjects (N 1,2,3,4,5) of each group (N = normals; LFe = left focal epilepsy; RFe = right focal epilepsy, Ge = generalized epilepsy) are illustrated. *Histograms:* log R/L value of the P300 amplitude in respect to zero (0) during the two types of stimulation (dotted: chord stimulation, striped: consonant stimulation). Higher algebraic ratio values during chords stimulation in respect to consonant stimulation are assumed as a right hemispheric engagement, while lower values are a left hemispheric engagement. *Chords and stop consonants* illustrate the types of stimulation. Stimuli are symbolized by deflections of the dotted and striped areas. From ref. [5].

The responses were evoked using six chords taken from an excerpt of a symphony (musical stimuli) and six stop consonants (b,d,g,p,c,k) were employed as verbal stimuli. The EEG power spectra were recorded while the subject was listening to a musical selection (musical stimuli) and a verbal passage (verbal stimuli).

The results suggest that: (1) in the normal subjects, the bioelectrical asymmetry is consistent with the nature of the stimulus, i.e. the musical stimuli induce a greater EEG engagement of the right hemisphere, whereas the verbal stimuli engage the left hemisphere to a greater extent; (2) the bioelectrical asymmetry is consistent with the nature of the stimulus also in the patients affected by primary generalized non convulsive epilepsy, but the hemispheric asymmetry appears to be lower than in normal subjects, as if the epileptic discharges were producing a 'noise effect' interfering with the recording of the bioelectrical phenomena under investigation; (3) in right and left focal epilepsy, a well-defined asymmetry was found in the EP recorded from the two hemispheres being higher in the hemisphere unaffected by the epileptic focus (fig. 3). This result indicates a preferential engagement of the normal hemisphere, regardless of its 'specialization', thus suggesting a role of functional replacement in information processing.

No changes in P300 latency were observed in any epileptic patients, thus suggesting that the epileptic functional focus does not interfere with the chronological processes of language processing.

Conclusions

In recent years there have been disputes about the theoretical bases of the electrophysiological approach to investigate the cognitive function, and criticism has been advanced against the results of investigations carried out by means of EEG processing. One of the most important reasons for such criticism is the wide spectrum of physiological and pathological changes which modify EEG parameters, particularly those considered functionally related to the unilateral or prevalent engagement of one hemisphere only. Despite this criticism, improvements in techniques and methods together with their consequent wider use have led to more data being accumulated.

Our research, summarized in the present paper, was carried out in order to verify whether certain experimental conditions are essential to the validity of techniques and methods employed to demonstrate hemispheric asymmetries by EEG processing.

The following points must be underlined:

(1) In normal subjects EEG power spectra and EP are reliable parameters capable of showing the selective engagement of one hemisphere using appropriate stimuli; during sleep, a functional hemispheric asymmetry is observed, the subject's mentation being an important factor in inducing

the prevalence of the right or left hemisphere. However, in SREM the right hemisphere was seen to prevail. Using a 1-c/deg grating as a visual stimulus in normal subjects, N1–P1 complex of EP shows a greater amplitude in the right hemisphere. The finding suggests that the visual lateralized processing occurs at the sensory level.

(2) In elderly cerebrovascular patients with CT mild brain atrophy but without any focal neurological symptom, there is greater prevalence of the alpha band in the right hemisphere, and the P300 latency is longer (without asymmetries) than in a control group of normal young people.

(3) In non-convulsive generalized epileptics the EEG power spectra and EP hemispheric asymmetries, induced by acoustic stimuli engaging one or the other hemisphere (verbal or musical stimuli), were similar to those in normal subjects, but of lower amplitude. In partial complex epilepsies a prevalence of the same EEG parameters was found in the unaffected hemisphere, irrespective of the two different kinds of stimulation.

(4) Our positive findings, obtained when investigating normal subjects, elderly patients with mild cerebrovascular disease and epileptics, demonstrate how EEG power spectra and EP can be used as parameters to study different functional activities of the two hemispheres both in normal and abnormal brains. The different stimuli used in each kind of investigation and the condition of awakeness or sleep, under which the experiments were carried out, suggest that better results are obtained when the methods include an appropriate combination of the kind of the stimulus and the processed EEG parameter explored in a certain cortical area. In general the combination of more than one parameter is a mean (or a more complete mean) of demonstrating hemispheric asymmetries.

References

1 Angeleri, F.; Marchesi, G.F.; Provinciali, L.; Scarpino, O.: Umiltà, C.: Studio della P300 durante somministrazione di un test discriminativo visuo-motorio in soggetti con atrofia cerebrale. Riv. It. Elettroencef. Neurofisiol. Clin. 3: 293–305 (1978).

2 Angeleri, F.; Provinciali, L.; Scarpino, O.; Signorino, M.: EEG spectral analysis, P300 and CNV in bilateral parieto-temporal areas during single and contemporary intermittent verbal task: a clinical approach. Res. Commun. Psychol. Psychiat. Behav. 7: 86–96 (1982).

3 Angeleri, F.; Scarpino, O.; Signorino, M.: Information processing and hemispheric specialization: electrophysiological study during wakefulness, stage 2 and stage REM sleep. Res. Commun. Psychol. Psychiat. Behav. 9: 121–138 (1984).

4   Angeleri, F.; Signorino, M.; Scarpino, O.; Provinciali, L.: Indici elettrofisiologici e neurofisiologici della dominanza emisferica nell'epilessia. Boll. Lega It. Epil. *45/46:* 191–198 (1984).
5   Angeleri, F.; Signorino, M.; Scarpino, O.; Provinciali, L.: Hemispheric specialization in generalized and partial epilepsy. A study of asymmetry of P300 and alpha power spectra during selective acoustic stimulation. Res. Commun. Psychol. Psychiat. *12:* 33–53 (1987).
6   Barrett, G.; Blumhart, L.D.; Halliday, A.M.; Halliday, E.; Kriss, A.: A paradox in the lateralization of the visual evoked response. Nature *261:* 253–255 (1976).
7   Begleiter, H.: Evoked brain potentials and behavior (Plenum Press, New York 1979).
8   Berlucchi, G.: Una ipotesi neurofisiologica sulle asimmetrie funzionali degli emisferi cerebrali nell'uomo; in Angeli, Umiltà, Neuropsicologia Sperimentale; pp. 95–120 (Riviste, Milano 1982).
9   Bigum, H.B.; Dustman, R.E.; Beck, E.C.: Visual and somatosensory evoked responses from mongoloid and normal children. Electroencef. Neurofisiol. Clin. *3:* 293–305 (1970).
10 Bradshaw, J.L.; Gates, A.; Patterson, K.: Hemispheric differences in processing visual patterns. Q. Jl exp. Psychol. *28:* 595–606 (1967).
11 Bradshaw, J.; Nettleton, N.C.: The nature of hemispheric specialization in man. Behav. Brain Sci. *4:* 51–91 (1981).
12 Butler, S.R.; Glass, A.: Asymmetries in the CNV over left and right hemispheres while subjects await numeric information. Biol. Psychiat. *2:* 1–16 (1974).
13 Callaway, E.; Harris, P.R.: Coupling between cortical potentials from different areas. Science *183:* 873–875 (1974).
14 Chartok, H.E.; Glassman, P.R.; Poon, L.W.; Marsh, G.R.: Changes in alpha rhythm asymmetry during learning of verbal and visuospatial tasks. Physiol. Behav. *15:* 237–239 (1975).
15 Cohen, G.: Hemisphere differences in serial versus parallel processing. J. exp. Psychol. *87:* 349–356 (1973).
16 Denes, F.; Umiltà, C.: I due cervelli. Neuropsicologia dei processi cognitivi (Mulino, Bologna 1978).
17 Desmedt, J.E.: Scalp recorded cerebral event related potentials in man as point of entry into the analysis of cognitive processing; in Schmidt, The organization of the cerebral cortex (MIT Press, Cambridge 1981).
18 Donchin, E.; McCarthy, G.; Kutas, M.: Electroencephalographic investigation of hemispheric specialization; in Desmedt, Language and hemispheric specialization in man: cerebral ERPs. Prog. clin. Neurophysiol., vol. 3, pp. 212–242 (Karger, Basel 1977).
19 Foulkes, D.; Pope, R.: Primary visual experience and secondary cognitive elaboration in stage REM: a modest confirmation and extension. Percept. Mot. Skills *37:* 107–118 (1973).
20 Friedman, D.; Simson, R.; Ritter, W.; Rapin, I.: Critical evoked potentials elicited by real speech words and human sounds. Electroenceph. clin. Neurophysiol. *38:* 13–19 (1975).
21 Galbraith, G.C.; Squires, N.; Altair, D.; Gliddon, J.B.: Electrophysiological assessment in mentally retarded individuals: from brainstem to cortex; in Begleiter, Evoked potentials and behavior, pp. 229–245 (Plenum Press, New York 1979).

22   Galin, D.; Ornstein, R.: Lateral specialization of cognitive mode: an EEG study. Psychophysiology 9: 412–418 (1972).

23   Geschwind, N.; Levitsky, W.: Human brain: left-right asymmetries in temporal speech region. Science 161: 186–187 (1968).

24   Gevins, A.S.; Doyle, J.C.; Schaffer, R.E.; Kallaway, E.; Yeager, C.: Lateralized cognitive processes and the electroencephalogram. Science 207: 1005–1008 (1980).

25   Giannitrapani, D.: Developing concepts of lateralization of cerebral functions. Cortex 3: 353–370 (1967).

26   Giannitrapani, D.: EEG changes under differing auditory stimulations. Archs gen. Psychiat. 23: 445–453 (1970).

27   Giannitrapani, D.: Scanning mechanisms and the EEG. Electroenceph. clin. Neurophysiol. 30: 139–146 (1971).

28   Giannitrapani, D.; Kayton, L.: Schizophrenia and EEG spectral analysis. Electroenceph. clin. Neurophysiol. 36: 377–386 (1974).

29   Giannitrapani, D.: Spectral analysis of the EEG; in Dolce, Kunkel, Computerized EEG analysis, pp. 384–492 (Fischer, Stuttgart 1975).

30   Giannitrapani, D.: Laterality preference, electrophysiology and the Brain. Electromyogr. clin. Neurophysiol. 19: 105–123 (1979).

31   Giannitrapani, D.: Spatial organization of the EEG in normal and schizophrenic subjects. Electromyogr. clin. Neurophysiol. 19: 125–145 (1979).

32   Giannitrapani, D.: Localization of language and arithmetic functions via EEG factor analysis. Res. Commun. Psychol. Psychiat. Behav. 7: 39–55 (1982).

33   Giannitrapani, D.: The electrophysiology of intellectual functions (Karger, Basel 1985).

34   Goldstein, L.; Stolzfus, N.W.; Gardocki, J.F.: Changes in interhemispheric amplitude relationships in the EEG during sleep. Physiol. Behav. 8: 811–815 (1972).

35   Goldstein, L.; Harnad, S.R.: Quantitated EEG correlates of normal and abnormal interhemispheric relations; in Desmedt, Language and hemispheric specialization in man: cerebral ERPs. Prog. clin. Neurophysiol., vol. 3, pp. 161–171 (Karger, Basel 1977).

36   Goodin, D.S.; Squires, K.C.; Starr, A.: Long latency event related components of the auditory evoked potential in dementia. Brain 10: 635–648 (1978).

37   Goodin, D.S.; Waltz, D.A.; Aminoff, M.J.: Task-dependent hemisphere asymmetries of the visual evoked potential. Neurology 35: 378–384 (1985).

38   Grunau, R.V.E.; Purves, S.J.; McBurney, A.K.; Low, M.D.: Identifying academic aptitude in adolescent children by psychological testing and EEG spectral analysis. Neuropsychologia 19: 79–86 (1981).

39   Kinsbourne, M.: Mechanisms of hemispheric interaction in man; in Kinsbourne, Smith, Hemispheric disconnection and cerebral function, pp. 260–285 (Thomas, Springfield 1974).

40   Kutas, M.; Hillyard, S.A.: Event-related potentials in cognitive science; in Gazzaniga, Handbook of cognitive neuroscience, pp. 387–490 (Plenum Press, New York 1984).

41   Lehmann, D.: Fluctuations of functional state: EEG patterns, and perceptual and cognitive strategies; in Koukku, Lehmann, Angst, Functional states of the brain: their determinants, pp. 189–202 (Elsevier, North-Holland Biomedical Press, Amsterdam 1980).

42   Liberson, W.T.; Fried, P.: EEG power spectrum and confusion in the elderly. Electromyogr. clin. Neurophysiol. *21:* 253–367 (1981).

43   Matsumiya, Y.; Tagliasco, P.; Lombroso, C.T.; Goodglass, H.: Auditory evoked response: meaningfulness of stimuli and interhemispheric asymmetry. Science *175:* 790–792 (1972).

44   Morgan, A.H.; McDonald, P.G.; McDonald, H.: Differences in bilateral alpha activity as a function of experimental task with a note on lateral eye movement and hypnotizability. Neuropsychologia *9:* 459–469 (1971).

45   Murri, L.; Stefanini, A.; Navona, C.; Dominici, L.; Muratorio, A.; Goldstein, C.: Automatic analysis of the hemispheric EEG relationship during wakefulness and sleep. Res. Commun. Psychol. Psychiat. Behav. *9:* 121–138 (1982).

46   Rhodes, L.E.; Dustman, R.E.; Beck, E.C.: The visual evoked response: a comparison of bright and dull children. Electroenceph. clin. Neurophysiol. *27:* 364–372 (1969).

47   Scheibel, A.B.: A dendritic correlate of human speech; in Geschwind, Galaburda, Cerebral dominance: the biological foundations, pp. 43–53 (Harvard University Press, Cambridge 1984).

48   Semmes, J.: Hemispheric specialization: a possible clue in mechanisms. Neuropsychologia *6:* 11–26 (1968).

49   Sergent, J.: Role of the input in visual hemispheric asymmetries. Psychol. Bull. *93:* 481–512 (1983).

50   Shucard, D.W.; Cummins, K.R.; Thomas, D.G.; Shucard, J.L.: Evoked potentials to auditory probes as indices of cerebral specialization of function. Replication and extension. Electroenceph. clin. Neurophysiol. *52:* 389–393 (1981).

51   Signorino, M.; Provinciali, L.; Ceravolo, G.; Chiaramoni, L.; Angeleri, F.: Hemispheric specialization for visuo-spatial stimuli: preliminary results of an evoked potential approach; in Gallai, Maturation of the CNS and evoked potentials; Excerpta Med. Int. Congr. Ser., No. 714, pp. 413–418 (1986).

52   Sperry, R.W.: Lateral specialization of cerebral function in the surgically separated hemispheres; in McGuigam, Schoonover, The psychophysiology of thinking (Academic Press, New York 1973).

53   Teuber, H.L.: Why two brains? in Schmitt, Worden, The neurosciences: third study program (MIT Press, Cambridge 1974).

54   Wood, C.C.: Average evoked potentials and phonetic processing in speech perception; in Desmedt, Language and hemispheric specialization in man: cerebral ERPs. Prog. clin. Neurophysiol., vol. 3, pp. 73–86 (Karger, Basel 1977).

55   Yingling, C.D.: Lateralization of cortical copuling during complex verbal and spatial behaviors; in Desmedt, Language and hemispheric specialization in man: cerebral ERPs. Prog. clin. Neurophysiol., vol. 3, pp. 151–160 (Karger, Basel 1977).

Prof. Franco Angeleri, MD, Clinica Neurologica dell'Università di Ancona,
I-60100 Torrette di Ancona (Italy)

Giannitrapani, Murri (eds.), The EEG of Mental Activities,
pp. 136–148 (Karger, Basel 1988)

EEG Characteristics of Frontal Midline Theta Activity

Tsuyoshi Inouye, Tsutomu Ishihara, Kazuhiro Shinosaki, Seigo Toi, Satoshi Ukai

Department of Neuropsychiatry, Osaka University Medical School, Osaka, Japan

Frontal midline theta activity (Fmθ) is a train of rhythmic waves at the frequency of 6–7 Hz which has a focal distribution with a maximum around the frontal midline. The train usually lasts for more than 1 s and tends to wax and wane [14, 27]. Fmθ can be induced particularly by the performance of a mental task.

Theta activity at the midline of the frontal area during rest and sleep has been considered to be a nonspecific abnormal rather than completely normal pattern [21, 24, 25]. This activity seems to correspond with Fmθ. In normal subjects, however, Fmθ can be observed during rest, a mental task and sleep (stages 1 and REM) although its occurrence during rest and sleep is relatively rare [13]. Fmθ thus can be considered to be a normal pattern even if Fmθ can be observed in such cerebral disorders as epilepsy. There is an interindividual variability in Fmθ occurrence [14, 18]. The incidence of Fmθ during a mental task in a normal population is 32–73%, although this percentage varies with age [27].

Fmθ during a mental task reflects a particular mental state which cannot be clearly defined. Although Fmθ can occur in various mental tasks (e.g. mental arithmetic, tracing a maze, counting the number of cubes piled up in a 3-dimensional representation, imagining a scene), it is necessary to concentrate on their tasks during a longer period of time [12, 14]. A sustained state of increased selective attention seems to be a necessary, though not sufficient, condition for the occurrence of Fmθ. Mizuki et al. [19] have reported that the appearance of Fmθ during a mental task has a periodicity of 20–290 s, suggesting that the periodicity reflects a fluctuation of attentive state. $Fm\theta$ can be more frequently induced after a biofeedback training [26].

$Fm\theta$ often has a notching at a fixed point in the ascending or descending phase for each wave [8]. Furthermore, delta activity at a frequency close to half that of $Fm\theta$ is sometimes seen during $Fm\theta$ occurrence. These waveforms suggest the presence of the harmonic and subharmonic components of $Fm\theta$ [9, 10]. The aim of this paper is to describe the EEG characteristics of $Fm\theta$ by use of various EEG analysis methods in order to study the generation mechanisms of $Fm\theta$.

Methods

Five normal male subjects with well defined $Fm\theta$ during the performance of a mental task for more than 5 s were studied. Their ages ranged from 16 to 18 years. They sat at a desk in an electrically shielded and sound-proofed room and were instructed to perform a Uchida-Kraepelin test for 5–10 min. The Uchida-Kraepelin test consists of adding 2 adjacent numbers and writing down the last of the added 2-digit number.

EEG were recorded from 13 electrodes placed at F_{p1}, F_{pz}, F_{p2}, $F_{pz}-F_z'$, F_3, F_3-F_z', F_z, F_z-F_4', F_4 F_z-C_z', C_3, C_z and C_4, each referenced to a linked ear. The soft sign (') indicates an intermediate position between neighboring electrodes of the 10–20 system. The 13 EEG channels were digitized at a sampling interval of 4.8 ms for 4.91 s during the appearance of $Fm\theta$. EEG were low-pass filtered (40 Hz cut-off, down 24 dB at 50 Hz) to avoid aliasing. One to 3 artifact-free epochs were obtained for each subject. In some cases, EEG recordings were made only on paper from electrode locations other than the 13.

The power spectrum for each electrode location was estimated by use of the fast Fourier transform (FFT) for each epoch. One epoch was divided into 4 segments. Each segment was tapered with a 10% cosine taper. The power spectral values were averaged over the 4 consecutive segments and smoothed by a Hanning window. The frequency resolution was 0.82 Hz.

The cross spectrum was estimated for the electrode pairs from an antero-posterior midline row: F_{pz} and $F_{pz}-F_z'$, $F_{pz}-F_z'$ and F_z, F_z and F_z-C_z' and F_z-C_z' and C_z and for the electrode pairs from a transverse row across F_z: F_3 and F_3-F_z', F_3-F_z' and F_z, F_z and F_4-F_z', F_4-F_z' and F_4. The phase spectrum and the coherence function were calculated from the cross spectrum for each pair.

The bispectrum was estimated at F_{pz}, F_3, F_z, F_4 and C_z to confirm that the frequency components half and twice the frequency of $Fm\theta$ are the first subharmonic and the first harmonic components which are phase-locked to $Fm\theta$ (for the detailed procedures of computation, see Huber et al., [6]). In the same way as the computation of power spectrum, the bispectra were averaged across the 4 consecutive segments and a Hanning window was applied to the power spectrum. The bicoherence (normalized bispectrum) was calculated from the bispectrum. The first subharmonic and the first harmonic components were judged to be present if the bicoherence values were significant at the 95% confidence level.

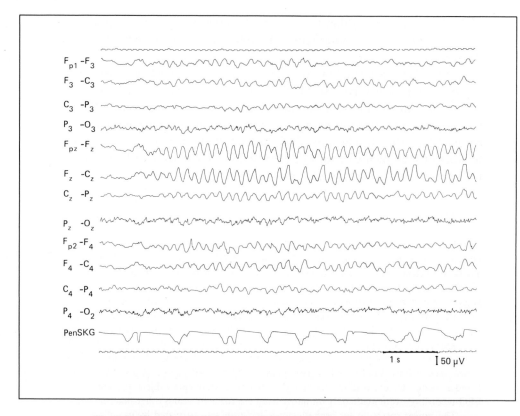

Fig. 1. Fmθ during Uchida-Kraepelin test. 50–80 μV rhythmic theta activity at 6.5 Hz occurs predominantly around F_z during the Uchida-Kraepelin test. 5 s after the start of the task, the train of Fmθ appeared and continued for about 7 s in this subject. The frequency and amplitude of alpha activity in parieto-occipital regions are unrelated to the occurrence of Fmθ.

Topographic mappings for Fmθ and its first subharmonic and harmonic components were obtained from the square root of the power (in μV). Equipotential lines were interpolated between electrodes with spline function.

Chronotopogram was obtained to describe the spatio-temporal relationships of Fmθ and its subharmonic component in both an antero-posterior midline and a transverse row across F_z. EEG were passed through 2 digital filters (one with stopband cutoff frequencies of 1 and 5 Hz and passband cutoff frequencies of 2.5 and 4.5 Hz and another with stopband cutoff frequencies of 4.5 and 8 Hz and passband cutoff frequencies of 5 and 7 Hz), separately for delta and theta activity. The amplitudes at every 4.8 ms were interpolated between electrodes with spline function.

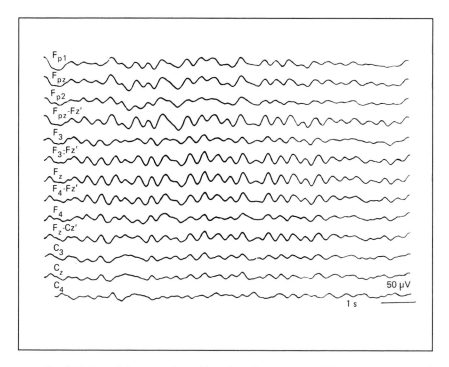

Fig. 2. Delta activity at prefrontal locations. Large delta activity with a notching of various amplitudes is intermixed with Fmθ predominantly at prefrontal midline locations during Fmθ occurrence. A delta wave with a larger notching cannot be differentiated from 2 theta waves.

Results

Fmθ during the Uchida-Kraepelin Test

50–100 μV rhythmic theta activity at 6.5 Hz appeared predominantly at F_z during the Uchida-Kraepelin test in all subjects (fig. 1). Five to 10 s after the start of the task, the train of Fmθ usually appeared and continued for 2–20 s while waxing and waning. The amplitude and frequency of alpha activity at parieto-occipital areas were not related to the appearance of Fmθ. Large delta activity occurred mainly at prefrontal locations (i.e. F_{p1}, F_{pz} and F_{p2}) with a notching in 2 subjects as shown in figure 2. As the notching had various amplitudes, one delta wave with a larger notching could not be differentiated from 2 theta waves.

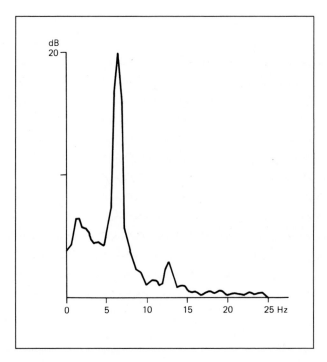

Fig. 3. Power spectrum of Fmθ. A prominent peak at 6.5 Hz and 2 smaller peaks at 3.2 and 13.0 Hz are seen at F_z in the power spectrum. The ordinate indicates the power in dB and the abscissa the frequency in Hz.

Power Spectrum

A prominent peak at 6.5 Hz and smaller peaks at 3.2 and 13.0 Hz were usually seen in most locations in the power spectrum (fig. 3). The peak frequency of Fmθ was 6.5 Hz in all epochs and subjects. The 6.5-Hz frequency component was largest at F_z while the 3.2-Hz frequency component was largest at F_{pz} in 2 subjects. The delta frequency of 3.2 Hz was almost half the theta, and the beta frequency of 13.0 Hz was twice the theta.

Cross Spectrum

The phase difference at 6.5 Hz for each pair was averaged over 2 or 3 epochs except in 2 subjects. In an antero-posterior midline row, the mean phase differences at 6.5 Hz averaged across 5 subjects between F_{pz} and

Table I. Phase differences of Fmθ in an antero-posterior midline row across F_z

Subject	$F_{pz}-F_{pz}-F_z'$	$F_{pz}-F_z'-F_z$	$F_z-F_z-C_z'$	$F_z-C_z'-C_z$
1	+8.5	+8.9	+9.9	+7.5
2	+0.3	+3.7	+2.7	+2.4
3	+28.7	−0.5	+0.4	−7.7
4	+1.6	+0.3	−0.3	+4.0
5	+4.7	+1.5	+12.4	+23.8
Mean	+8.8	+2.8	+5.0	+6.0
SD	10.4	3.8	5.8	11.4

Phase differences are expressed in degrees. The sign + indicates an anterior phase lead and the sign − a posterior phase lead. Mean and SD are shown below.

Table II. Phase differences of Fmθ in a transverse row across F_z

Subject	$F_3-F_3-F_z'$	$F_3-F_z'-F_z$	$F_z-F_4-F_z'$	$F_4-F_z'-F_4$	F_3-F_z	F_4-F_z	F_3-F_4
1	+14.0	+11.5	+2.5	+4.9	+25.9	+7.3	+16.8
2	+12.0	+10.6	+5.0	+6.9	+22.6	+11.7	+7.8
3	+12.5	+5.0	+0.3	+14.3	+17.5	+14.9	+2.3
4	+21.7	+2.2	+4.5	+16.7	+24.5	+21.5	+2.5
5	+14.5	+5.1	−2.9	+8.3	+21.3	+4.8	+20.3
Mean	+14.9	+6.9	+1.9	+10.2	+22.4	+12.0	+9.9
SD	4.1	4.0	3.2	5.1	2.9	6.7	8.3

The sign + indicates a lateral phase lead, and the sign − a midline phase lead.

$F_{pz}-F_z'$, $F_{pz}-F_z'$ and F_z, F_z and F_z-C_z' and F_z-C_z' and C_z were +8.8, +2.8, +5.0 and +6.0, respectively (the sign + indicates an anterior phase lead, table I). In a transverse row across F_z, the mean phase differences averaged at 6.5 Hz across 5 subjects between F_3 and F_3-F_z', F_3-F_z' and F_z, F_z and F_z-F_4', F_z-F_4' and F_4, F_3 and F_z, F_4 and F_z and F_3 and F_4 were +14.9, +6.9, +1.9, +10.2, +22.4, +12.0 and +9.9, respectively (the sign + indicates a lateral phase lead, table II). The mean phase difference between F_3 and F_4 (i.e. between most lateral locations in the transverse row) was smaller than between either F_3 or F_4 and F_z. The coherence values at the peak

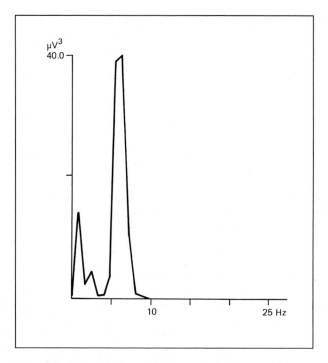

Fig. 4. Bispectrum of Fmθ at 6.5 Hz. A prominent peak at 6.5 Hz is seen at 6.5 Hz in the bispectrum at F$_z$. The coherence value is significant at the 95% confidence level. The ordinate indicates the power in μV^3 and the abscissa the frequency in Hz.

frequency of Fmθ were above 0.80. The directions of phase differences show prefrontal and lateral leading, indicating that Fmθ at midline locations occurred later than in prefrontal and lateral locations.

Bispectrum

The bispectrum at 6.5 Hz showed a prominent peak at 6.5 Hz in most locations (fig. 4). The bicoherence value between the 2 frequencies was significant at the 95% confidence level. This indicates that the 6.5 Hz frequency component was the first harmonic component of Fmθ. The bispectrum at 3.2 Hz showed a significant peak at 3.2 Hz mostly in prefrontal areas, indicating that the first subharmonic component occurred more frequently. The second subharmonics and harmonics as well as the third were sometimes found.

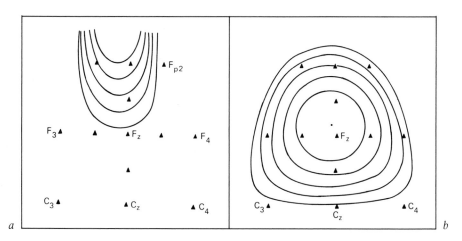

Fig. 5. Topographical mapping of Fmθ and its first subharmonic component. An elliptical distribution of Fmθ is seen to have a maximum just anterior to F_z with the long axis longitudinally and the short axis transversely *(b)*. The first subharmonic component had a distribution with a maximum just anterior to F_z *(a)*. Equipotential lines are interpolated between electrodes with spline function in steps of 15 *(b)* and 40 μV *(a)*. The triangle indicates the position of each of 13 electrodes.

Topographic Mapping

An eliptical distribution of Fmθ was found to have a maximum either just anterior to F_z (i.e. F_{pz}–F_z') or F_z with the long axis longitudinal and the short axis transverse (fig. 5b). The first subharmonic component had a distribution with a maximum just anterior to F_{pz} (fig. 5a). These maxima were not exactly at the midline in 2 subjects, as in figure 5. The distribution of the first harmonic component did not markedly differ from that of Fmθ.

Chronotopogram

Negative and positive maxima immediately anterior and lateral to F_z or at F_z remained almost stationary, though slightly changed with time, in an antero-posterior midline and a transverse row in all epochs and subjects. In a transverse row, smaller amplitude Fmθ occurred earlier at lateral locations (e.g. F_3 and F_4) and then larger amplitude Fmθ at F_z (fig. 6). In an antero-posterior midline row, Fmθ appeared earlier at prefrontal locations (e.g. F_{pz}, fig. 7). These time relationships agreed well with the results of the phase spectrum.

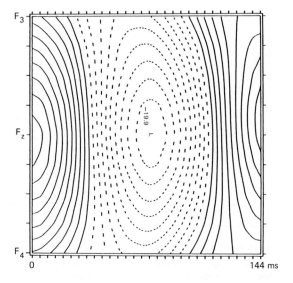

Fig. 6. Chronotoprogram of Fmθ in a transverse row across F_z. One negative and 2 positive waves are shown. Their maxima are at F_z. Fmθ occurs earlier at lateral locations. The amplitude of maps is plotted as a function of time (in abscissa) and space (electrode location in ordinate). The time base is 144 ms. The electrode location is from F_3 (top) to F_4 (bottom) in a transverse row. Broken lines indicate negative and solid positive. Equipotential lines are interpolated between electrodes with spline function in steps of 12 μV.

Discussion

Fmθ and its harmonically related components were distributed predominantly in frontal and prefrontal areas. These areas may be anatomically and functionally related to the appearance of Fmθ. The prefrontal areas are assumed to be involved in thought process [7, 29] and in focusing and resistance to intrusion of unrelated stimuli [4]. It, therefore, seems that the active performance of a mental task is likely to induce Fmθ in the prefrontal and frontal areas.

Eye movement artifacts are often found in the EEG in these areas. Giannitrapani [4] has pointed out a possibility that Fmθ is eye movement artifacts. This possibility can be ruled out by the differences between the 2 potentials in dominant frequency, waveforms and distribution and rhythmicity, because eye movement potentials with eyes open during a mental task usually have a scalp distribution with a maximum anterior to prefron-

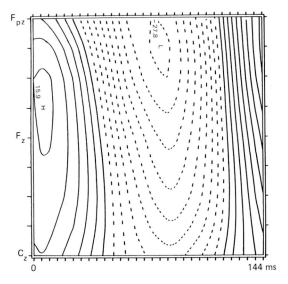

Fig. 7. Chronotopogram of Fmθ in an antero-posterior midline row. One negative wave and 2 positive waves are shown in an antero-posterior midline row. Their maxima are seen anterior to F_z. Fmθ occurs earlier at prefrontal locations. The ordinate indicates the locations from F_{pz} (top) to C_z (bottom) in an antero-posterior midline row and the abscissa the time. The time base is 144 ms. Equipotential lines are interpolated between electrodes in steps of 6 μV with spline function.

tal areas, a dominant frequency of less than 6 Hz, irregular waveforms and little or no harmonics.

Fmθ spread in the directions of both from anterior to posterior areas and from lateral to medial areas in the prefrontal, frontal and central regions over the scalp. It could not be determined precisely whether overall directions are from anterior to midline areas, because the phase relationships and the chronotopograms were examined only from an antero-posterior midline and a transverse row across F_z. The direction of spread of EEG activity has been described as being highly complicated because an earlier occurrence in the areas remote from a maximum area has been reported in such EEG activities as alpha rhythm and seizure discharges [5, 11, 17, 22]. Further, since beneath the scalp at the frontal midline a longitudinal fissure separates the 2 hemispheres, this anatomy should be taken into consideration in discussing the distribution and spread direction of Fmθ on the scalp. At the midline the scalp distribution may not reflect directly a potential field in the cortex. This potential field in each hemisphere is possibly located slightly lateral to the midline. The scalp distribution at the midline may seem to be the summation of the bilateral potentials of the same polarity which reaches a maximum at the time when Fmθ spreads to the midline. This phenomenon is compatible with the suggestion that auditory evoked potential and pattern reversal visual evoked potential at the midline are the algebraic sum of bilateral potentials [2, 23].

The 2 potential fields of Fmθ can be considered to be mutually interconnected possibly by either the corpus callosum or the midline subcortical structures which causes the simultaneous occurrence of the bilateral fields. A phase difference of 9.9 degrees between F_3 and F_4 (i.e. most distant electrode pairs across F_z) at 6.5 Hz corresponds with 4.2 ms (table II). This interhemispheric delay time of Fmθ is too short to explain the transcallosal transmission because the conduction time has been reported to be about 10 ms [16]. Particularly in subjects 3 and 4, the potentials at F_3 and F_4 can be considered to occur synchronously because the interhemispheric delay time of Fmθ was about 1 ms. The probable connection, therefore, seems to be the midline subcortical structures by which Fmθ is triggered to spread to the cortical areas in both hemispheres at the same time.

In this Fmθ generating model there are 2 major locations, one in the cortical area slightly lateral to the midline for each hemisphere and another in the midline subcortical structures. The possible propagation sequence is as follows: the midline subcortical structures, lateral prefrontal and medial frontal areas for each hemisphere. It seems that the origin of Fmθ is not necessarily in the midline subcortical structures in this model because these areas may make a feedback loop between the cortical areas and the midline subcortical structures.

Such EEG activities as sleep spindle, transient sharp wave, frontal intermittent delta activity, midline spike, 3 Hz spike and wave and P300 show a midline maximum. It has been suggested that the midline subcortical structures, particularly the thalamus, play an important role in the genesis of these activities [1, 3, 15, 20, 28, 29]. The same might be true for Fmθ generation.

The mechanism of generating subharmonics and harmonics in the EEG remains unclear. The first subharmonic component of Fmθ appeared more frequently in prefrontal areas than in fronto-central areas. Therefore, this subharmonic component (i.e. delta activity) has a prominent area in the prefrontal. In regard to the subharmonic component, the occurrence of

Fmθ seems to be differently modified by different cortical areas in the antero-posterior direction.

Fmθ during a mental task might be heterogeneous during sleep because there is no psychophysiological relationship between the 2 states. However, the morphology and the distribution of Fmθ during a mental task are similar to those during sleep although the distribution of Fmθ shifts slightly toward central areas (i.e. between F_z and C_z) from wakefulness to sleep [13]. In one subject whose sleep recording could be made, the first harmonic component of Fmθ became larger in a drowsy state, as in the finding of White and Tharp [25] that a 6.5–8.5 Hz rhythmic activity localized in frontal areas has larger harmonic components during the transition from wakefulness to sleep. The sleep spindle at 13 Hz also appeared with the same scalp distribution as the harmonic component. The generation mechanism of Fmθ harmonics may be influenced by arousal level. Further investigations will be required for clarifying a relationship between Fmθ and the sleep spindle.

References

1 Andersen, P.; Andersson S.A.: Thalamic origin of cortical rhythmic activity; in Remonds, Handbook of electroencephalography and clinical neurophysiology, vol. 2C, pp. 90–118 (Elsevier, Amsterdam 1974).

2 Blumenhardt, L.D.; Halliday, A.M.; Hemispheric contributions to the composition of the pattern-evoked potential waveform. Exp. Brain Res. 36: 53–69 (1982).

3 Ehle, A.; Schenley, C.; Jones, M.G.: Clinical correlates of midline spikes. An analysis of 21 patients. Achs Neurol. 38: 355–357 (1981).

4 Giannitrapani, D.: The electrophysiology of intellectual functions (Karger, Basel 1985).

5 Gottman, J.: Measurement of small time differences between EEG channels. Electroenceph. clin. Neurophysiol. 56: 501–514 (1983).

6 Huber, P.J.; Kleiner, B.; Gasser, T.; Dumermuth, G.: Statistical methods for investigating phase relations in stationary stochastic processes. IEEE Trans. Audioacoustics AU-19: 78–86 (1971).

7 Ingvar, D.H.; Philipson, L.: Distribution of cerebral blood flow in the dominant hemisphere during motor ideation and motor performance. Ann. Neurol. 2: 230–237 (1977).

8 Inouye, T.; Ishihara, T.; Shinosaki, K.; Generating mechanism for frontal midline theta activity (in Japanese). Rinsho Noha/Clin. Electroenceph. 26: 796–798 (1984).

9 Inouye, T.; Ishihara, T.; Shinosaki, K.: Harmonics and subharmonics of frontal midline theta activity (in Japanese). Rinsho Noha/Clin. Electroenceph. 27: 377–380 (1985).

10 Inouye, T.; Ishihara, T.; Shinosaki, K.; Toi, S.: Distribution of the subharmonics of frontal midline theta activity (in Japanese). Rinsho Noha/Clin. Electroenceph. *27:* 501–505 (1985).
11 Inouye, T.; Shinosaki, K.; Yagasaki, A.: The direction of spread of alpha activity over the scalp. Electroenceph. clin. Neurophysiol. *55:* 290–300 (1983).
12 Ishihara, T.; Izumi, M.: Fmθ and imaginative mental activities (in Japanese). Rinsho Noha/Clin. Electroenceph. *6:* 381–384 (1975).
13 Ishihara, T.; Izumi, M.: Distribution of the Fmθ on the scalp in mental calculation, resting and drowsy states (in Japanese). Rinsho Noha/Clin Electroenceph. *18:* 638–644 (1976).
14 Ishihara, T.; Yoshii, N.: Multivariate analytic study of EEG and mental activity in juvenile delinquents. Electroenceph. clin Neurophysiol. *33:* 71–80 (1972).
15 Jankel, W.R.; Niedermeyer, E.: Sleep spindles. J. clin. Neurophysiol. *2:* 1–35 (1985).
16 Lemieux, J.F.; Blume, W.: Topographical evolution of spike-wave complexes. Brain Res. *373:* 275–287 (1986).
17 Mars, N.J.I.; Lopes da Silva, F.H.: Propagation of seizure activity in kindled dogs. Electroenceph. clin. Neurophysiol. *56:* 194–209 (1983).
18 Mizuki, Y.; Tanaka, M.; Isogaki, H.; Nishijima, H.; Inanaga, K.: Fmθ and personality. Jap. J. EEG EMG *4:* 182–191 (1976).
19 Mizuki, Y.; Tanaka, M.; Isogaki, H.; Nishijima, H.; Inanaga, K.: Periodic appearances of theta rhythm in the frontal midline area during performance of a mental task. Electroenceph. clin. Neurophysiol. *49:* 345–351 (1980).
20 Nelson, K.R.; Brenner, R.P.; Paz, D. de la: Midline spikes. EEG and clinical features. Archs Neurol. *40:* 473–476 (1983).
21 Palmer, F.B.; Yarwoth, S.; Niedermeyer, E.: Frontal midline theta rhythm. Clin. Electroenceph. *7:* 131–138 (1976).
22 Petsche, H.; Pockberger, H.; Rappelsberger, P.: On the search for the sources of the electroencephalogram. Neuroscience *11:* 1–27 (1984).
23 Vaughan, H.G., Jr.; Ritter, W.: The sources of auditory evoked responses recorded from the human scalp. Electroenceph. clin. Neurophysiol. *28:* 360–367 (1970).
24 Westmoreland, B.F.; Klass, D.W.: Midline theta rhythm. Archs Neurol. *43:* 139–141 (1986).
25 White, J.C.; Tharp, B.R.: An arousal pattern in children with organic cerebral dysfunction. Electroenceph. clin. Neurophysiol. *37:* 265–268 (1974).
26 Yamaguchi, Y.; Niwa, K.; Feedback training and self-control of frontal theta burst of EEG appearing during mental work (in Japanese). J. Jap. Psychosom. Soc. *14:* 344–353 (1974).
27 Yamaguchi, Y.: Frontal midline theta rhythm (in Japanese). Rinsho Noha/Clin. Electroenceph. *25:* 276–281 (1983).
28 Yingling, C.D.; Hosobuchi, Y.: A subcortical correlate of P300 in man. Electroenceph. clin. Neurophysiol. *59:* 72–76 (1984).
29 Zurek, R.; Delgado, J.S.; Froescher, W.; Niedermeyer, E.: Frontal intermittent rhythmical delta activity and anterior bradyrhythmia. Clin. Electroenceph. *16:* 1–10 (1985).

T. Inouye, MD, Department of Neuropsychiatry,
Osaka University Medical School, Fukushima-ku, Osaka 553 (Japan)

Giannitrapani, Murri (eds.), The EEG of Mental Activities,
pp. 149–152 (Karger, Basel 1988)

The Role of 13-Hz Activity in Mentation

Duilio Giannitrapani

Veterans Administration Medical Center, Perry Point, Md., USA

The earliest investigators in EEG, including Berger in 1938 [Gloor, 1969], hypothesized that cognitive functions could be detected through electrocortical functions based on the notion that mental activity is consequent to organized neural activity with its chemical and electrophysiological correlates. The nature of this organization is discussed here.

EEG history shows that alpha activity (8–12 Hz) became the first target primarily because it was the dominant rhythm of the brain, and it was easily scorable by visual inspection of the tracing. In light of the inconsistent findings obtained, a broad frequency search was undertaken to determine whether specific frequencies relate to intellectual functions. A brief account of Giannitrapani's [1972, 1985] work is followed by a current interpretation.

The range of frequencies studied was from 1 to 32 Hz. Every 8 s 16 power values were obtained via BMDX92 [Massey and Jennrich, 1969], one for each of 16 frequency bands each 2 Hz wide. To determine the topography of these functions, 16 scalp positions were studied concomitantly for a total of 256 spectral values. The values of one EEG sample for each of 8 conditions were averaged so that spectral scores represented 64 s of EEG. The matrix of EEG power spectral scores consisted of 16 frequency bands × 16 brain areas. Each of these EEG values was correlated (Spearman rhos) with each of the 11 subtest scores and the 3 main IQ test scores of the WISC (Wechsler Intelligence Scale for Children) which had been obtained for each of the 11- to 13-year-old subjects (n = 56) who were non-VA normal volunteers from the Chicago area.

The single frequency with the greatest correlatability between steady-state EEG spectral scores and intellectual scores was the 13-Hz band which included activity from 12 to 14 Hz. Significant correlations of this band were preponderant among all WISC Verbal subtests and, in addition, in

		Frequency bands														
		1	3	5	7	9	11	13	15	17	19	21	23	25	27	29	31
Prefrontal	left														•		
	right																
Lat. frontal	left						•	●									
	right						●	•									
Frontal	left						•	●	•		•	•	•				
	right			•		•	•	■	•	•		•					
Central	left						•	●	•								
	right	•					•	■	•				•				
Temporal	left						•	●									
	right						•	●									
Post-temporal	left							•									
	right						•										
Parietal	left						•	●		•			•				
	right						•	●									
Occipital	left						•	•					•				
	right																

• Rho with p < 0.05 (0.26–0.34); ● rho with p < 0.01 (0.35–0.42); ● rho with p < 0.001 (0.43–0.48); ■ rho with p < 0.0001 (> 0.48). A minus (–) preceding the dot indicates a negative rho.

Fig. 1. Significant Spearman rhos between WISC Full Scale IQ scores and 64 s of EEG power (n = 56).

the Block Design subtest. The remainder of the Performance subtests showed only a few vestiges of this significant activity.

Figure 1 shows the significant correlations present in the matrix of Spearman rhos obtained between each of the frequency components of 64 s of EEG and WISC Full IQ scores. Evident are significant correlations in the 13-Hz band which overshadow the significant correlations in all other frequencies. The 13-Hz band is not to be confused with EEG-dominant activity which was investigated in previous EEG-intellectual function studies. The 13-Hz activity has an amplitude many times smaller than dominant alpha activity which for this group was represented in the power of the 11-Hz band. Furthermore, the strongest correlations are in central areas which do not contain particularly strong amplitudes in dominant alpha activity, the latter being characteristic of parietal and occipital areas.

In this study, dominant activity shows some relationship with intellectual functions as demonstrated by the strength of significant correlations in the 11-Hz band. Among the Verbal subtests these correlations are stronger than in the 13-Hz band only in the Information subtest matrix and are absent in the Arithmetic subtest. They are also absent from the Performance subtests except for a small vestige in Block Design.

The earlier hypothesis that alpha activity was a correlate of intellectual functions finds therefore some statistical support in the present findings. It appears to relate to the portion of verbal activity which is dependent on old funds of knowledge. It does not represent leakage from the 13-Hz activity because of the diversity of the distribution mentioned above. It is to be emphasized that the correlations in the 11-Hz band are weaker than in the 13-Hz band in spite of the fact that the amplitude is many times greater. The 13-Hz correlations are strongest in the Comprehension subtest, attesting to some role it must have in facilitating conceptual ability.

A function as hierarchically complex and phylogenetically recent as intelligence, however, should not be expected to be mediated by a unidimensional structure such as a single frequency band. Our own research indicated that low beta activity seems to serve an organizing role such as in the case of the Comprehension, Arithmetic and Picture Arrangement subtests (see Giannitrapani and Collins [this vol.], figures 2, 3 and 4). One of the several conditions needed for performing mental tasks may be the interaction between several scanning mechanisms postulated by Giannitrapani [1971], based on Eccles' [1951] formulation. Eccles explained how alpha activity at around 10 Hz can be based on the circulation of impulses in closed self-reexciting neuronal chains. It follows that with higher cortical excitation levels the neurons would be excited with greater frequency. The theoretical limit of frequencies generated by closed self-reexciting chains would be about 66 Hz [Giannitrapani, 1985].

What we might be observing in the matrices of correlations between intellectual tasks and EEG is the activity produced in a myriad of such self-reexciting chains. Since the EEGs used in this study are unrelated to the intellectual task in question, it can be postulated that the strength of these circuits is related to their availability for performing an intellectual task in proportion to their regularity which permits better synchronization between neuronal chains and therefore a more predictable, more efficient and faster transfer of information.

The strongest correlations between intellectual functions and 13-Hz activity always occur in the central areas. Even though scalp locations show great variation with cortical structures, the central electrode placement can be thought of as overlying the premotor area which is vaguely associated with motor functions. Luria [1966], however, ascribed to this area a more specific intellectual function. He observed that lesions in this area were related to intellectual deficits concerned with the inability to synthesize and automate mental activity.

This area can be thought of also as including the one described by Eccles and Robinson [1984] in which impulses appear prior to the initiation of movement and obstensibly prior to the appearance of impulses anywhere else in the brain. They concluded that the supplementary motor area is the closest neurophysiological evidence of mind. There seems to be an integrative role being served by the central areas, a role which has not been apparent in traditional studies such as cortical stimulation, lesion studies or traditional neuropsychology.

References

Eccles, J.C.: Interpretation of action potentials evoked in the cerebral cortex. Electroenceph. clin. Neurophysiol. *3:* 449–464 (1951).
Eccles, J.C.; Robinson, D.N.: The wonder of being human (Free Press, New York 1984).
Giannitrapani, D.: Scanning mechanisms and the EEG. Electroenceph. clin. Neurophysiol. *30:* 139–146 (1971).
Giannitrapani, D.: EEG correlates of intellectual functioning. Abstract Guide XXth Int. Congress of Psychology, Tokyo, August 1972, p. 493 (Science Council of Japan, Tokyo 1972).
Giannitrapani, D.: The electrophysiology of intellectual functions (Karger, Basel 1985).
Gloor, P.: Hans Berger on the electroencephalogram of man. Electroenceph. clin. Neurophysiol., suppl. 28 (1969).
Luria, A.R.: Higher cortical functions in man (Basic Books, New York 1966).
Massey, F., III; Jennrich, R.: BMDX92: time series spectrum estimation; in Dixon, BMD biomedical computer programs, X series, pp. 193–224 (University of California Press, Berkeley 1969).

Duilio Giannitrapani, PhD, Veterans Administration Medical Center, PO Box 193, Perry Point, MD 21902 (USA)

Giannitrapani, Murri (eds.), The EEG of Mental Activities,
pp. 153–168 (Karger, Basel 1988)

Focused Arousal, 40-Hz EEG, and Motor Programming

Jon DeFrance[a], *Daniel E. Sheer*[b]

[a] Department of Neurobiology and Anatomy, University of Texas Medical School,
[b] Department of Psychology, University of Houston, Houston, Tex., USA

In a seminal paper on the neural mechanisms of serial ordering in behavior, Lashley [12] addressed problems concerning the syntax of motor action which are directly relevant today. In elegantly detailed examples of motor patterning, he came to the conclusion that such programming could not be explained by sensory control or by the simple association of specific segmental units. Rather, he proposed that ...

'Consideration of rhythmic activity and of spatial orientation forces the conclusion, I believe, that there exists in the nervous organization elaborate systems of interrelated neurons capable of imposing certain types of integration upon a large number of widely spaced effector elements; in the one case transmitting temporally spaced waves of facilitative excitation to all effector elements; in the other, imparting a directional polarization to both receptor and effector elements ... It is probably not far from the truth to say that every nerve cell of the cerebral cortex is involved in thousands of different reactions. The cortex must be regarded as a great network of reverberatory circuits constantly active. A new stimulus, reaching such a system, does not excite an isolated reflex path but must produce widespread changes in the pattern of excitation throughout a whole system of already interacting neurons ... The space coordinate system and various types of set or priming may be pictured as patterns of subthreshold facilitation pervading the network of neurons which is activated by the more specific external stimulus' [12, pp. 127, 131, and 134].

In the past 35 years there has been much progress in detailing the operation of interconnected brain regions in motor programming and performance. These have included, in various integrative actions: the premotor, supplementary motor, and primary motor areas [2, 16, 17]; limbic, prefrontal, and parietal areas [13, 16]; the basal ganglia [4], and the cerebellum [11]. Evarts et al. [6], using unit analysis, have gone on to identify centrally stored, prestructured sets of muscle commands. However, the problems posed by Lashley for the syntax of motor action still remain largely unanswered.

A psychological construct of focused arousal has been developed in considerable detail as a first-order functional component in attention [22, 25]. As a basic, simple system of interactive brain function with properties proposed by Lashley, this construct may be equally important in motor programming.

The neural substrate for focused arousal involves phasic arousal circuitry, whose major source of ascending cholinergic pathways from the brain stem is the parabrachial nucleus, extending from the level of the genu of the facial nerve caudally to the level of the trochlear nucleus rostrally. From here a prominent distribution, traveling through the lateral hypothalamus, goes to the basal forebrain, including the caudateputamen, accumbens and also the substantia innominata which distributes to the cortex. Another pathway from the brain stem also projects to the cortex where dense terminal fields are found in layers V and VI. Another prominent distribution goes to the nucleus reticularis of the thalamus and the thalamic relay nuclei, including the lateral geniculate and medical geniculate bodies. With efferent and modulatory descending pathways from limbic structures and cortex, particularly frontal cortex, and limbic interconnections, this is the phasic arousal system, the focal neural substrate for the facilitation of focused arousal in specific sensory and motor circuitry. Focused arousal itself is the facilitated – momentarily coherent – specific sensory and motor circuitry [22].

Focused arousal interactive with stimulus sets serves an energizing function of selective specificity. This selective specificity is expressed in the physical measurement operation as distinctive spatial amplitude patterns of coherent resonance at an optimal periodicity in relevant sensory and motor circuitry (40-Hz EEG). Using the olfactory bulb as a model and nonlinear dynamics theory, Freeman [7] and Freeman and Skarda [8] have detailed the neural mechanisms for selective specificity in the relatively simple neural substrate of the olfactory bulb. Distinctive spatial amplitude patterns of 40-Hz oscillations replicated across the bulb convey specific odor information.

We can generalize the neural mechanisms beyond the olfactory bulb without, of course, the elegant detail that Freeman [7] has worked out for the bulb. Spatial amplitude patterns of coherent oscillations are determined by unique templates of synaptic connections, forming – with focusing behavioral operations such as reinforcement contingencies – distinctive nerve cell assemblies for discriminative information.

The specificity of the information conveyed is determined by the distinctive spatial pattern of unit cell specificities, defined by the modulatory controlled specific content of the sensory input – stimulus sets. The energy that momentarily fixes the unique spatial pattern at a significantly high amplitude level is the coherent resonance – focused arousal. It is the configurational property of the unit specificities – ensembles of interconnected neurons replicated across relevant circuitry – that is distinctive, and not individual units which are involved in multiple patterns. Also, any individual unit may or may not enter into a specific organized pattern from time to time.

For this higher-order functional component – focused arousal interactive with stimulus sets – the 40-Hz EEG acts as a carrier frequency. The 40-Hz EEG is short-hand notation for different high-frequency EEG bands in the gamma range which index the optimal periodicity for different species [1, 24]. In humans, the optimal frequency band is 36–44 Hz [23].

In the present study, the 40-Hz EEG measurement operation of focused arousal will be used to examine its functioning in motor programming and performance. Forty-Hz EEG will be recorded bilaterally from the motor cortex and parietal-temporal-occipital (PTO) cortex during a series of reaction-time tasks. Three sets of reaction-time tasks, performed by normal adults, have been designed to be maximally sensitive to motor programming differences. A complex-choice reaction-time (CCRT) task consists of trials in which the subject knows he will have to respond versus trials in which he knows he will not have to respond. A variable probability reaction-time (VPRT) task consists of trials in which the subject has an 80% response probability versus trials in which he has a 20% probability of responding. A simple-choice reaction-time (SCRT) task consists of trials in which the subject responds on every trial. The results with these tasks will be discussed in terms of the neural dynamics of the 40-Hz EEG in motor programming.

Method

Subjects. Thirteen right-handed medical students served as subjects. All were in good health and free from obvious neurological disorders.

Equipment. The equipment used in this study included a microprocessor (Apple IIe) interfaced with a special-purpose 40-Hz detection unit [15, 20, 22], and a reaction-time module (Frederick Haer & Co.). The special-purpose 40-Hz detection unit was used to analyze EEG activity within a 40-Hz band (36–44 Hz).

The reaction-time module contained four LED lights (red, green, yellow, and white) and a button that the subject was to push in response to the appropriate light. The microprocessor controlled the presentation of the stimuli, recorded and stored the reaction time values, and synchronized the data collection from the 40-Hz detection module.

EEG Recording and Analysis. EEG electrodes were located according to the International 10–20 System. EEG activity was recorded bilaterally over the motor area (1 cm anterior to C3 and C2) and the parietal-temporal-occipital area (center of the O1-P3-T5 and O2-P4-T6 triangles). These electrodes were referenced to an electrode located at Cz, with a ground electrode over the nasion. The electrodes, of the disc variety (Grass Instrument Co.), were applied to the scalp with EC2 Electrode cream. They were tested just prior to recording to ensure impedances of less than 5kΩ.

There are serious problems encountered in trying to reliably record short, aperiodic bursts of 40 Hz from the human scalp. One is the greater attenuation of the higher frequency part of the EEG spectrum as it is volume-conducted to the electrodes. This reduces the absolute amplitude of the 40 Hz, generated from a restricted neuronal assembly, to a still lower level. Another problem is the frequency overlap of the 40-Hz with the higher amplitude of the EMG from the scalp muscles, which actually go down to 14 Hz but show a considerable increase in power above 30 Hz across a broad spectrum to 100 Hz and above. What is needed to overcome these difficulties are critical scalp electrode placements, considerable signal preprocessing, and 'state-of-the-art' special-purpose computer technology. Techniques for carrying out these objectives have been evolving [20–22]. The present procedure for recording 40-Hz EEG, concurrently with focusing behavioral operations, consists of a special-purpose computer, with analog and digital filter capability, master control, and user interface sections [15].

Signal preprocessing takes the form of a high-pass cutoff at 20 Hz and a low-pass cutoff at 90 Hz with a sharp 60-Hz notch filter. The control for muscle artifact depends on the broad-frequency spectrum of muscle, and an algorithm based on covariance analysis. EEG activity in the one-third octave range of 36–44 Hz with a center at 40 Hz is specified as uncorrected 40 Hz (Σy^2), and activity in the one-third octave window of 62–78 Hz with a center frequency at 70 Hz is specified as muscle (Σx^2). The corrected power function $\Sigma y'^2 = \Sigma y^2 - \Sigma xy^2$ represents the power of the 40-Hz EEG independent of muscle. The two electrode placements go first to two commercial bioamplifiers with high common mode rejection specifications. Dual outputs from the amplifiers go to a dual-beam oscilloscope for monitoring and to the digital filter section of the computer.

The digital filter section consists of a series of Intel 2920 analog microprocessors. The 2920 included A/D converters on the chip and is designed for high-speed signal processing applications. The 2920 first digitize the two input channels, and then implement bandpass filters and other detection algorithms to determine the presence of 40- and 70-Hz bursts which are then rectified to provide peaks (2x cycles). The 2920 work independently and give their results to the master control section.

The master control section consists of a single Intel 8751 microprocessor. The 8751 is a fast single-chip microprocessor with RAM, EPROM, I/O ports, timers, and a serial port all on the chip. The 8751 receives the results from the digital filter section for each channel, left and right, calculates the muscle algorithm and presents the final results through the user interface section.

The user interface section consists of an eight-channel thermal printer, a keyboard, and an eight-character display. The user is able to specify operating parameters, such as, threshold levels, number of cycles, duration of epochs, and start and stop computer analysis manually and by remote control. The thermal printer provides a printout of the final results. The entire system is packaged together with its own power supply.

The eight-channel thermal printer, for each designated epoch, prints out the following for both the left (L) and right (R) hemispheres: uncorrected 40-Hz peak power (Σy^2); 70-Hz peak power (Σx^2); number of 70-Hz peaks; corrected 40-Hz peak power ($\Sigma y'^2$) and corrected number of 40 Hz peaks (N). Mean peak powers

$$\frac{\Sigma y'^2}{N}$$

and normalized asymmetries

$$\frac{L-R}{L+R}$$

for both corrected 40-Hz peak powers and number of peaks can be calculated for each epoch. In this study, the measure of 40-Hz EEG activity used was the number of peak counts from the left and right hemispheres.

Reaction-Time Procedure. The behavioral protocol consisted of three different tasks, utilizing dominant-hand reaction time as the performance measure. The reaction time was defined as the time from the onset of the 'imperative' correct stimulus to the button press.

The three tasks were CCRT, VPRT, and SCRT. A trial in each task consisted of the initial presentation of a preparatory or ready stimulus (red light), followed by an imperative stimulus (green or yellow light). The offset of the preparatory and the onset of the imperative stimuli defined the preparatory interval. All three tasks were programmed with a constant preparatory interval of 12 s.

The EEG activity for these reaction time tasks was recorded only during the preparatory intervals, defined either by the offset of the preparatory stimulus (red light) and the onset of the correct stimulus (yellow or green light), or by the offset of the preparatory stimulus and the onset of an incorrect stimulus.

The CCRT task consisted of 20 trials. In this task, a correct response was possible when a certain stimulus combination appeared over two trials. For example, the subject was instructed to push the button to the yellow light only after a trial with a green light. A three-trial practice session was used to demonstrate this task. Because the previous trial always indicated if the subject was to respond on a subsequent trial, the 20 trials in this task could be divided into two groups of response trials (RESP) and no response trials (NRESP). The EEG peak counts were summed for each group of 10 trials for each subject. The instruction to the subjects were as follows:

'The red light is going to come on. It is going to tell you that either a green or yellow light will follow. You are not to press to the green, only the yellow...but, you are to press to the yellow only if the previous trial had a green light in it. If you press to the yellow light after the green light comes on then you will earn a point and the white light will come on to tell you that you have done it correctly. You are not to press to the green light, or the yellow light in any trial unless it follows a trial where a green light appears. Any questions?'

The VPRT task consisted of 30 trials. For this task, the instructions for trials 1–15 were as follows:

'In this task, the warning signal will again be a red light. The red light will come on to warn you that a yellow light may follow. For any given trial, there will be 8 chances out of 10 that the yellow light will follow the red light. When it does, you are to quickly press the button. But, in 2 chances out of 10, a green light will come on after the red light. When the green light comes on, you are not to press. Any questions?'

The instructions for trials 16–30 were as follows:

'Now we're going to change things on you. The red light will again come on to tell you that a yellow light may follow, but this time a yellow light will come on only 2 chances out of 10, and the green light will come on 8 chances out of 10. You're still to press the button to the yellow light, but now it will come on only 2 times out of 10. Any questions?'

The SCRT task consisted of 20 trials. The instructions to the subjects were as follows:

'Now, a red light will come on to warn you that either a green or yellow light will come on in one of two columns. I want you to press the button as soon as either the green or yellow light comes on, regardless of the column in which it appears. Press the button as soon as a green or yellow light comes on.'

The reaction time tasks were presented in the following sequence: complex-choise, variable probability, and simple choice. This complex to simple sequence was used to minimize a vigilance decrement over time.

Results

Reliable EEG data, free from muscle artifact, were obtained consistently across tasks in a group of 13 subjects, except for 2 cases. Subject No. 12 in the VPRT task had too much muscle artifact in motor cortex and subject No. 4 in the SCRT task also had too much muscle artifact in motor cortex. These 2 cases were included in the sample, but their EEG data on these two tasks were omitted from the summary measures and statistical analyses. Due to the wide range and nonnormal distributions of peak count scores for each subject on each task, the medians of these distributions were selected to best represent the summary measures of 40-Hz EEG peak counts for each subject on each of the groups of trials across the tree tasks.

These measures are shown in table I for the CCRT task, in table II for the VPRT task, and in table III for the SCRT task. These reaction-time tasks and, particularly, the experimental operations using these tasks – response trials versus nonresponse trials on the CCRT task and 80% response probability trials versus 20% response probability trials on the VPRT task – were carried out to make them maximally sensitive to motor cortex function. These tasks are not maximally sensitive to lateralized higher-order sensory-cognitive functions. In this way, the left and right PTO cortical EEG activity acts as a control for the results obtained with motor cortex.

On the CCRT task (table I), there is a significant difference on 40-Hz EEG peak counts with PTO cortex between left and right hemispheres on response trials. There are no other significant differences with the PTO cortex. The CCRT task was the most cognitively complex, effortful reaction-time task of the group of three, which may account for the left PTO cortex lateralization of 40-Hz EEG activity on this task.

With motor cortex on this CCRT task, there is clear, consistent left hemisphere lateralization of the 40-Hz peak counts, indexing right-handed motor programming and performance. There is a significant difference between the RESP and NRESP trials for the left hemisphere but not the right hemisphere and significant differences between LH and RH for both RESP and NRESP trials.

On the VPRT task, table II, none of the differences between distributions with PTO cortex are significant. With motor cortex on this VPRT task, there is again clear, consistent left hemisphere lateralization of motor cortex reflecting right-handed performance. There are significant differences between the 40-Hz peak counts in left hemisphere versus right hemisphere on both 80% probability trials and 20% probability trials. There is also a significant difference in the left hemisphere between 80% response probability trials versus 20% probability trials, but not in the right hemisphere.

On the SCRT task, table III, there are the same findings of no lateralization of 40-Hz EEG peak counts with PTO cortex, but a significant difference between left and right hemispheres in the motor cortex.

Table I. Median number of 40-Hz peak counts per subject, from the motor (MC) and PTO cortices of the left (LH) and right (RH) hemispheres during the performance of the CCRT task. This task was analyzed in terms of RESP and NRESP trials

Subject	PTO				MC			
	LH		RH		LH		RH	
	RESP	NRESP	RESP	NRESP	RESP	NRESP	RESP	NRESP
1	94	101	49	60	162	126	90	79
2	52	40	43	43	22	12	15	12
3	169	150	83	79	85	89	19	23
4	39	35	22	26	91	50	56	39
5	36	52	83	79	85	36	21	30
6	27	26	12	14	31	23	19	12
7	40	30	23	20	28	12	12	13
8	94	103	39	37	59	52	46	42
9	52	74	51	50	84	85	88	72
10	99	91	132	97	73	62	55	52
11	75	67	63	41	42	32	24	23
12	54	55	44	95	41	29	27	40
13	122	110	109	121	92	77	67	42
Mean	73.3	71.8	57.9	59.4[1]	66.0	52.7	41.5	36.8[2]
SD	41.0	37.2	35.2	33.7	38.1	34.0	27.5	21.5

[1] Differences between the distributions of the LH and RH for the RESP trials were significant beyond the 0.05 level on the Wilcoxon signed-ranks test. All other comparisons between RESP and NRESP and between RH and LH distributions were not significant.

[2] Differences between the distributions of the LH and RH for both the RESP and NRESP trials and between the RESP and NRESP for the LH were significant beyond the 0.05 level on the Wilcoxon signed-ranks test. The difference between the RESP and NRESP trials for the RH was not significant.

For ease of understanding, these overall findings are graphically represented in figure 1 for the PTO cortex and in figure 2 for the motor cortex. The ordinate in these figures are the means of the median distributions of the 13 subjects for each of the trial groupings with the different tasks. With PTO cortex, the only significant difference is between left and right hemisphere with the RESP trials on the CCRT tasks. The other differences are small and insignificant.

Table II. Median number of 40-Hz peak counts per subject, from the MC and PTO cortices of the LH and RH during the performance of the VPRT task. This task was analyzed in terms of 80% response probability trials and 20% response probability trials

Subject	PTO				MC			
	LH		RH		LH		RH	
	80%	20%	80%	20%	80%	20%	80%	20%
1	110	35	116	112	164	136	87	88
2	45	46	36	38	17	9	13	9
3	115	116	77	69	96	48	22	16
4	75	61	32	27	64	57	47	54
5	26	21	94	89	40	28	53	50
6	32	10	21	5	20	11	20	9
7	34	28	34	41	30	20	20	18
8	66	45	79	68	41	24	39	46
9	39	65	18	73	122	91	102	91
10	93	76	118	134	69	40	40	24
11	77	77	32	27	15	12	12	6
12	60	41	45	46				
13	38	40	24	18	60	61	42	42
Mean	62.3	50.9	55.9	57.5[1]	61.5	44.8	41.4	37.8[2]
SD	30.1	28.1	36.2	37.5	45.9	37.8	28.4	29.5

[1] None of the comparisons between RH and LH and 80 and 20% distributions were significant on the Wilcoxon signed-ranks test.
[2] Differences between the distributions of the LH and RH for both the 80 and 20% probability trials and between the 80 and 20% trials for the LH were significant beyond the 0.05 level on the Wilcoxon signed-ranks test. The difference between the 80 and 20% for the RH was not significant.

With motor cortex, there are large and significant differences between left and right hemispheres on all trial groupings – RESP trials and NRESP trials on the CCRT task, 80% response probability trials and 20% response probability trials on the VPRT task, and 100% response trials on the SCRT task. With the left hemisphere of the motor cortex, there are also significant differences on the RESP trials versus NRESP trials and on the 80% response probability trials versus the 20% response probability trials.

Table III. Median number of 40-Hz peak counts per subject, from the MC and PTO cortices of the LH and RH during the performance of the SCRT task

Subject	PTO		MC	
	LH	RH	LH	RH
1	72	73	153	85
2	59	19	14	15
3	151	95	43	12
4	44	18		
5	23	88	42	44
6	44	6	24	5
7	35	41	12	16
8	94	73	43	39
9	45	57	114	101
10	124	99	56	37
11	43	41	22	17
12	40	48	18	13
13	36	50	96	52
Mean	62.3	54.5[1]	53.1	36.3[2]
SD	38.3	30.0	44.9	30.5

[1] The difference between the LH and RH was not significant.
[2] The difference between LH and RH was significant beyond the 0.05 level with the Wilcoxon signed-ranks test.

All of these results with the motor cortex provide a consistent pattern of left hemisphere lateralization of right-handed motor programming and performance as indexed by 40-Hz EEG activity.

Discussion

The results of this study are quite clear and consistent. The 40-Hz EEG activity indexes the lateralized operation of focused arousal in motor programming – in the left motor cortex with a right-handed preparatory motor set to respond in reaction-time tasks. It is specified as motor programming rather than performance because the significant increases in

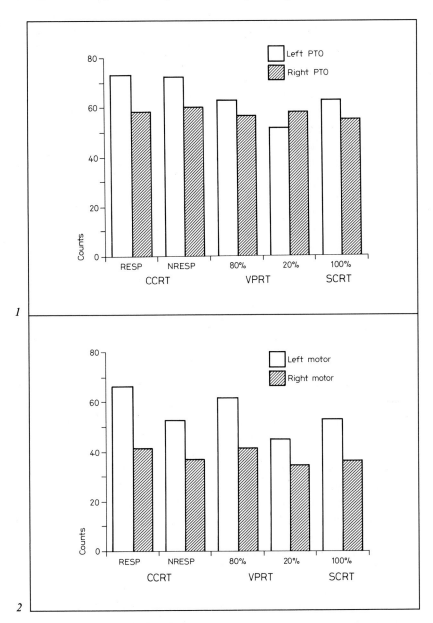

Fig. 1. Mean number of 40-Hz peak counts from the left and right PTO cortex for the CCRT, VPRT, and SCRT tasks (n = 13 subjects).

Fig. 2. Mean number of 40-Hz peak counts from the left and right motor cortex for the CCRT, VPRT, and SCRT tasks (n = 13 subjects).

40-Hz activity occurred between the warning signal and the imperative stimulus, just before the response. Further, levels of this EEG activity in the left hemisphere was significantly changed by behavioral operations which signal different probabilities of having to make a response – RESP trials versus NRESP trials on the CCRT task and 80% response probability trials versus 20% response probability trials on the VPRT task. This left hemisphere lateralization with right-handed motor activity has also been demonstrated with measures of cerebral blood flow [18] and with the terminal contingent negative variation (CNV) potentials and the readiness potentials (RP) [9].

This study also provides further data on the dissociation between 40-Hz EEG activity and muscle artifact in the same frequency band. In right-handed individuals, particularly when preparing to respond, there is higher muscle activity on the right side as compared with the left [19, 20]. On all 3 reaction-time tasks, there were consistently higher levels of EEG activity from the motor cortex on the left side. These significantly increased levels of 40-Hz EEG, associated with motor programming, was specific to the motor cortex locus because they did not occur in concurrent recordings from bilateral PTO cortex. On a wide range of sensory-cognitive processing tasks, there were significant lateralizations of the 40-Hz EEG from PTO cortex in both the left and right hemispheres with appropriate left and right tasks [reviewed in Sheer, 22]. The reaction-time tasks in this study were designed for maximal sensitivity to motor programming and minimal demands on sensory-cognitive processing so that the PTO cortical leads could serve as controls. These findings again emphasize the prime importance of having appropriate behavioral operations concomitant with recordings of electrical activities.

This study extends the operation of the first-order functional component, focused arousal, to the output side of cognitive processing and provides another measurement operation, 40-Hz EEG, in the investigation and analysis of higher-order motor functions, from the abstract plan of action [14] through the selection, sequencing and phasing of effector units [13]. The 40-Hz EEG is a particularly good analytic tool because it is a low-order functional component, a first-order interaction producing a simple system with a finite neural substrate and with some understanding of its neural dynamics. At neocortex the ascending cholinergic brain stem reticular system provides the steady background input to bias the level of depolarization in subsets of functionally connected cell assemblies. In the multisensory neocortex the biasing input of the ascending brain stem reticular system is multisensory, activated by collaterals into the brain stem reticular from the specific sensory systems.

Sensitivity in the form of neural gain depends on the level of depolarization bias as a consequence of steady background input. As cell assemblies become excited by background input, the neural gain increases, driving the neurons closer to their firing threshold. Hence, the probability of a subsequent signal input firing a neural response is increased. However, as sensitivity increases, there is a concomitant increase in instability. If numerous cells with excitatory connections were driven into a state of increased gain, an uninterrupted series of excitation would exist. One neuron would deliver an excitatory pulse to adjacent cells where it would stimulate neurons with heightened gain. This, in turn, would then feed back to the first cell, further increasing its excitatory gain. To prevent runaway excitation, inhibition of approximately equal magnitude interrupts the cycle of mutual excitation. This balance between excitatory and inhibitory influences provides system stability. The feedback loops resulting from mutually excitatory cell connections, mutually inhibitory connections, and excitatory-inhibitory interactions, i.e. recurrent inhibition, give rise to periodic oscillations recorded as EEG.

The coherent EEG reflects repetitive stimulation at a constant frequency for a limited time over a finite specific circuitry. The circuitry is defined behaviorally by focusing operations – the spatial-temporal patterning of sensory inputs, motor outputs, and reinforcement contingencies. Repetitive periodic excitation of cells maximizes the efficiency of synaptic transmission over the limited circuitry. Eccles [5] has well documented this property of frequency potentiation by demonstrating the maximal size of EPSP that develop with repetitive activation at different optimal frequencies for different neural networks.

The duration of repetitive periodic discharges at an optimal frequency is probably as significant in the transfer of information as the number and specificities of cells involved. Granit [10], in his quantitative studies on the control of tonic motor neurons of the spinal cord, concluded that frequency of firing was the main code determining rate of continuous discharge. Brookhart and Kubota [3] found a clear relationship between frequency of stimulation of the dorsal root and firing efficiency of motor cells in the spinal cord of frogs. At a frequency of 40/s the neurons behaved in a 'driven' fashion at a firing rate of unity, while below and above this frequency the firing pattern was more variable. For cortical pyramidal cells in cats, Stefanis and Jasper [28] found that their axon collaterals became particularly effective at relatively high frequencies of repetitive excitation. They also noted that the negative feedback of recurrent inhibition provides an automatic control on level of excitation – the greater the excitation, the more the feedback of inhibition.

A significant outcome of this loop – wherein recurrent inhibition sets up periodicity which sets up frequency potentiation – is the property of contrast. The negative feedback of recurrent inhibition particularly depresses those synapses that are weakly excited in the 'surround' and so serves to further shapen the focus of excitation. Behaviorally it is reflected, on the input side in focusing of attention on relevant stimuli and, on the output side, in greater precision of relevant movements. The operation of contrast as a function of surround inhibition has been detailed for spinal cord motor neurons [10], thalamocortical relay cells [5], and cortical motor cells [28].

A final point concerns the resonant property of the facilitated coherent circuitry. Singer [26] demonstrated that cellular networks within the visual cortex display properties of resonance ('ringing', a rhythmic discharge which persists after an input is removed) and hysteresis (a property of a system wherein it fails to return to baseline after an input is removed). These properties in cortical networks are facilitated by a central core of ascending cholinergic brain stem pathways. The firing patterns within their networks are analogous to distinct functional 'states', each of which is associated with a balance between excitatory and inhibitory influences. 'Any particular functional state tends to be stabilized by reverberation in positive feedback loops, aided by long time constants of inhibition' [26, p. 1105].

Singer et al. [27] have also demonstrated the importance of spatial-temporal contingencies in the cholinergic facilitation of visual cortex cells. 'An interesting phenomenon was the hysteresis in the facilitation of light responses. When the brain stem reticular formation stimulus was applied at the appropriate interval, it facilitated the light response over as long as 1 s and more. When, however, the conditioning stimulus was shifted by only 100 ms or less, it completely lost its facilitatory effect over the whole duration of the light stimulus. This suggests, first, that a precise timing between reticular activation and the initial transient component of the light response is necessary to obtain facilitation and, second, that once subliminal excitation has reached threshold, it becomes self-sustaining' [27, p. 87]. The 40-Hz EEG, coherent resonance at a optimal periodicity for maximal synaptic transmission over a finite circuitry, may thus be the 'temporally spaced waves of facilitative excitation to all effector units', which Lashley proposed for the syntax of action some 35 years ago.

Summary and Conclusions

A measurement operation, 40-Hz EEG, for a first-order functional component, focused arousal, was recorded from normal adults, bilaterally from motor cortex and parietal-temporal-occipital cortex, concomitant with motor programming and performance in a series of three reaction-time tasks. The 40-Hz EEG activity indexes the lateralized operation of focused arousal in motor programming – in the left motor cortex with a right-handed preparatory motor set to respond in these reaction-time tasks. This study extends the operation of the first-order functional component of focused arousal to the output side of cognitive processing and provides another measurement operation, 40-Hz EEG, in the investigation and analysis of higher-order motor function. A neural substrate for focused arousal was presented and the neural dynamics of its operation discussed. The 40-Hz EEG represents coherent resonance at an optimal periodicity for maximal synaptic transmission over a finite circuitry.

References

1   Bressler, S.C.; Freeman, W.J.: Frequency analysis of olfactory system EEG in cat, rabit, and rat. Electroenceph. clin. Neurophysiol. *50:* 19–24 (1980).
2   Brinkman, C.; Porter, R.: Supplementary motor area in the monkey: activity of neurons during performance of a learned motor task. Neurophysiology *42:* 681–709 (1979).
3   Brookhart, J.M.; Kubota, K.: Studies of the integrative function of the motor neuron; in Moruzzi et al., Brain mechanisms, vol. I, sect. 1, p. 38 (Elsevier, New York 1963).
4   De Long, M.R.; Georgopoulos, A.P.: Motor functions of the basal ganglia; in Handbook of physiology, sect. 1, vol. 1, p. 1017 (Am. Physiological Society, Washington 1981).
5   Eccles, J.C.: The physiology of synapses (Springer, New York 1964).
6   Evarts, E.V.; Shinoda, Y.; Wise, S.P.: Neurophysiological approaches to higher brain functions (Wiley, New York 1984).
7   Freeman, W.J.: Oscillatory potentials; in Sheer, Pribram, Attention: cognition, brain function, and clinical application (Academic Press, New York 1988).
8   Freeman, W.J.; Skarda, C.A.: Spatial EEG patterns, non-linear dynamics and perception: the neo-Sherrington view. Brain Res. Rev. *10:* 147–175 (1986).
9   Gaillard, A.W.K.: Cortical correlates of motor preparation; in Nickerson, Attention and performance, vol. VIII, p. 75 (Erlbaum, Hillsdale 1980).
10 Granit, R.: Recurrent inhibition as a mechanism of control; in Moruzzi et al., Brain mechanisms, vol I, p. 23 (Elsevier, New York 1963).
11 Ito, M.: The cerebellum and neural control (Raven Press, New York 1984).

12 Lashley, K.S.: The problem of serial order in behavior; in Jeffress, Cerebral mecha-
    nisms in behavior, p. 112 (Wiley, New York 1951).
13 Martenuik, R.G.; Mackenzie, C.C.: Information processing in movement organiza-
    tion and execution; in Nickerson, Attention and performance, vol. VIII, p. 29 (Erl-
    baum, Hillsdale 1980).
14 Miller, G.A.; Galantes, E.; Pribram, K.H.: Plans and the structure of behavior (Holt,
    New York 1960).
15 Raghavan, N.; Glover, J.R.; Sheer, D.E.: A microprocessor-based system for diagno-
    sis of cognitive dysfunction. IEEE Trans. biomed. Engng *10:* 942–948 (1986).
16 Roland, P.E.: Organization of motor control by normal human brain. Hum. Neuro-
    biol. *2:* 205–216 (1984).
17 Roland, P.E.; Larsen, B.; Lassen, N.A.; Skinhoj, E.: Supplementary motor area and
    other cortical areas in organization of voluntary movements in man. Neurophysiol-
    ogy *43:* 118–136 (1980).
18 Roland, P.E.; Meyer, E.; Shibasaki, T.; Yamamoto, Y.L.; Thompson, C.J.: Regional
    cerebral blood flow changes in cortex and basal ganglia during voluntary movements
    in normal human volunteers. Neurophysiology *48:* 467–480 (1982).
19 Sanders, A.F.: Some effects of instructed muscle tension on choice reaction and
    movement time; in Nickerson, Attention and performance, vol. VIII, p. 59 (Erl-
    baum, Hillsdale 1980).
20 Sheer, D.E.: Biofeedback training of 40 Hz EEG and behavior; in Kamiya et al.,
    Biofeedback and self-control 1976/1977. An annual review, p. 435 (Aldine, Chicago
    1977).
21 Sheer, D.E.: Focused arousal, 40 Hz EEG, and dysfunction; in Elbert et al., Self-
    regulation of the brain and behavior, p. 64 (Springer, Berlin 1984).
22 Sheer, D.E.: A working cognitive model of attention – to fit in the brain and in the
    clinic; in Sheer, Pribram, Attention: cognition, brain function, and clinical applica-
    tion (Academic Press, New York 1988).
23 Sheer, D.E.: Brain damage and dysfunctions; in Sheer, Pribram, Attention: cogni-
    tion, brain function, and clinical application (Academic Press, New York 1988).
24 Sheer, D.E.; Grandstaff, N.: Computer-analysis of electrical activity in the brain and
    its relation to behavior. Top. Probl. Psychiat. Neurol., vol. 10, pp. 160–172 (Karger,
    Basel 1970).
25 Sheer, D.E.; Schrock, B.: Attention; in Hannay, Experimental techniques in human
    neuropsychology, p. 95 (Oxford University Press, New York 1985).
26 Singer, W.: Center-core control of visual cortex function; in Schmit, Worden, The
    neurosciences: Fourth Study Program, p. 1093 (MIT Press, Cambridge 1979).
27 Singer, W.; Tretter, F.; Cynader, M.: The effect of reticular stimulation on sponta-
    neous evoked activity in the cat. Visual cortex. Brain Res. *102:* 71–90 (1976).
28 Stefanis, C.; Jasper, H.: Recurrent collateral inhibition in pyramidal tract neurons.
    Neurophysiology *27:* 855 (1964).

Jon DeFrance, PhD, Department of Neurobiology and Anatomy, University of
Texas Medical School, PO Box 20108, Houston, TX 17025 (USA)

Giannitrapani, Murri (eds.), The EEG of Mental Activities,
pp. 169–181 (Karger, Basel 1988)

EEG Correlates of Clinical Heterogeneity of Schizophrenia

Dargut Kemali, Silvana Galderisi, Mario Maj

Department of Medical Psychology and Psychiatry, First Medical School,
University of Naples, Naples, Italy

The EEG correlates of schizophrenic disorders have been the subject of a large amount of literature during the past five decades [1–3]. Several different patterns have been described (table I), but these data have been regarded as nonconclusive [4] and it has been stated that there is no EEG pattern characteristic of schizophrenia [5, 6]. Part of the above discrepancy might be interpreted as a consequence of the clinical and biological heterogeneity of schizophrenic disorders.

Quite recently, a dichotomous approach to the investigation of schizophrenia has been reproposed, mainly through the work of Crow [7] in England and Andreasen [8] in the USA.

According to Crow's model, schizophrenia includes two main syndromes: 'type I syndrome', also referred to as positive or florid schizophrenia, and 'type II syndrome', also indicated as negative or defect schizophrenia.

Type I syndrome would be characterized by positive symptoms (such as delusions and hallucinations) and responsiveness to neuroleptics; its pathogenesis has been linked to a hyperactivity of the mesolimbic dopaminergic system, on the basis of postmortem brain studies in which the density of D_2 dopamine receptors was found increased in limbic areas [9]. Type II syndrome would be marked by negative symptoms (flattened affect, alogia, avolition, etc.), a higher degree of cognitive impairment and a poor response to antipsychotic drugs. Both CT scan evidence of enlarged lateral ventricles [10, 11] and postmortem findings of neuronal loss, mainly in the temporal lobes [12], seem to support the hypothesis that

Table I. Different EEG patterns described in schizophrenic patients

General slowing and dysrhythmia [51, 52]
Decrease of alpha activity [53, 54]
Epileptic potentials [55, 56]
Choppy activity (sparse or no alpha and prominent, irregular fast beta activity) [6, 57]
Increased beta activity and reduced average alpha frequency [23]
Hypernormal EEG (regular, rhythmic, synchronized alpha rhythm) [50]
Increased theta activities [58]

atrophic changes in the brain represent the underlying damage in type II syndrome.

The above dichotomy has also been supported by biochemical findings of decreased cerebrospinal fluid (CSF) 5-hydroxy-indoleacetic acid [13], homovanillic acid and noradrenaline (NA) levels [14] in patients with enlarged ventricles, in contrast to the findings of increased CSF NA levels in paranoid schizophrenics [15].

Not very far from Crow's model, Andreasen's interpretation of the positive/negative dimension relies upon Jackson's notion [16] that positive symptoms reflect a release from higher cortical inhibitors, while negative aspects may be related to cortical atrophy.

In both Jackson's and Luria's model [17] of brain functioning, the higher cortical inhibitors would correspond to the frontal lobes.

Cerebral blood flow (CBF) and positron emission tomography (PET) studies in schizophrenic subjects have shown a relative reduction of activity in frontal regions [18], in particular in the prefrontal cortex [19], together with an increased activity in postcentral areas. This pattern is in contrast to both the normal one (hyperfrontality) and that of Alzheimer dementia. The lowest frontal CBF was found in patients with a more pronounced negative symptomatology and a correlation was observed between positive symptoms (i.e. hallucinations) and a decreasing CBF in frontal regions and an increasing flow postcentrally [20].

A dysfunction of the frontal lobes and of their influence on the basal ganglia and superior colliculus has also been proposed as the most likely explanation of saccadic intrusions in smooth pursuit eye movements observed in several schizophrenics, as well as of some neuropsychological findings [21].

To our knowledge, EEG correlates of the positive and negative aspects of schizophrenia and their relation to other biological variables have not been adequately explored. This is rather surprising, since different computerized EEG (C-EEG) aspects in chronic versus acute schizophrenia have been reported in the literature, with a diffuse EEG slowing or a hyperstable slow alpha rhythm in the former and an increase in the fast frequencies in the latter [22–24].

In this article, we will summarize the results of two investigations carried out by our group during the last 3 years [25, 26], designed to assess simultaneously several clinical, historical, biological and neuropsychological variables in schizophrenic subjects. The data obtained will be discussed in relation to findings provided by CT scan, CBF and PET studies, using Luria's systemic approach to the brain's functioning as a reference model.

Subjects and Methods

Study 1

In study 1, CSF catecholamines, platelet monoamine-oxidase (MAO) activity and variables of C-EEG were assessed in a sample of 20 patients (7 males and 13 females, aged 18–36 years) fulfilling Research Diagnostic Criteria [27] for acute schizophrenia.

The control populations consisted of 20 subjects without personal or family history of major psychoses (7 males and 13 females, aged 18–35 years), who required lumbar puncture as part of a diagnostic evaluation for suspected neurologic illness and, by the time of discharge, were determined to suffer from functional disease or not to be ill.

All subjects were placed on a low monoamine and alcohol-and caffeine-restricted diet. CSF samples were taken from schizophrenics and controls after a wash-out period of at least 15 days, according to the procedure described in Kemali et al. [15]. On the same day of lumbar puncture, patients underwent EEG recording, blood sampling for platelet MAO estimation and psychopathological evaluation (by means of the Comprehensive Psychopathological Rating Scale (CPRS) [28].

CSF NA, as well as dopamine (DA) and adrenaline, levels were assayed by the radioenzymatic method of Da Prada and Zurcher [29]. Platelet MAO activity was determined by the method of Wurtman and Axelrod [30] as modified by Winter et al. [31].

The C-EEG recording and analysis method has been described in detail elsewhere [32]. In brief, all the EEG were recorded at the same hour (8.00 a.m.). Six monopolar leads were used, according to the 10–20 system (A_1F_3; A_2F_4; A_1C_3; A_2C_4; A_1O_1; A_2O_2). A position encoder in binary numeration allowed the selection of 30 artifact-free epochs of 4 s. The EEG signal was stored on a 7-channel analog tape recorder and then transferred to a 1000 L Hewlett Packard computer through an analog to digital converter. The cut-off frequency was 64 Hz and the sampling interval 8 ms. Using a fast Fourier transform, the raw spectra were computed with a resolution of 0.25 Hz and then averaged. For further analysis, the spectra were divided into frequency bands: delta 2.25–3.75 Hz; theta 3.75–7.75 Hz; alpha 7.75–13.25 Hz; beta 13.25–31.75 Hz. For each frequency band, the following spectral descriptors were used: the relative activity (percent value of the EEG signal power), the barycentric frequency (average weighted frequency) and the barycentric radius (mean band width).

Statistical analysis was made by Student's t-test (comparison between CSF catechol-amine levels of schizophrenics and controls) and Pearson's correlation coefficient (evalu-ation of relationships between CSF NA levels and C-EEG parameters, CPRS scores and platelet MAO activity).

Study 2

CT scan was performed in a population of 50 patients fulfilling DSM III criteria [33] for schizophrenic disorder and a control group of 25 healthy subjects matched to patients for age, sex and educational level. Only subjects aged less than 40 years, with negative neurological examination and no history of organic brain disorders, ECT and insulin comas, were included in the study.

The CT scan procedure and the method for evaluating the area of the lateral ventri-cles are described in Kemali et al. [34]. Briefly, the area of the lateral ventricles was measured in the slice showing them at their largest and expressed as the percentage of the area of the inner table of the skull in the same slice. This percentage was called the ventricular brain ratio (VBR).

The mean VBR value was significantly higher in the schizophrenic sample than in the normal control group (4.52 ± 2.25 vs 3.37 ± 1.56, $p < 0.02$). Thirteen patients (26% of the sample) had VBR values more than 2 SD higher than the control group. They were classified as 'patients with enlarged ventricles'.

Only 21 of the 50 schizophrenic patients could undertake a 15-day wash-out period. They therefore became available for C-EEG investigation. The C-EEG procedure was the same as described above. During the same day of the EEG recording, all the patients were administered the CPRS and the Scale for the Assessment of Negative Symptoms [35]. Moreover, they were tested by the Premorbid Adjustment Scale [36] and by the Disability Assessment Schedule [37].

Univariate statistical analysis (comparison between patients with enlarged and nor-mal ventricles with respect to each variable) was performed by Student's t-test and χ^2 method with Yates' correction.

Results

Study 1

Mean CSF NA levels were found to be significantly increased in schizophrenics as compared with controls (150.2 ± 4.5 vs 131.8 ± 4.1 pg/ml, $p < 0.01$).

CSF NA levels were significantly correlated with C-EEG indicators of activation: a positive correlation with beta relative activity and alpha bary-centric frequency was observed in frontal and central leads and a negative correlation was found with alpha relative activity (table II). No significant correlation emerged between NA concentration and platelet MAO activity as well as CPRS symptom scores.

Table II. Correlation coefficients between CSF noradrenaline levels and C-EEG indicators of activation

C-EEG parameter	Correlation coefficient
Alpha relative activity	
Frontal R	−0.60***
Central R	−0.56**
Occipital R	−0.41
Frontal L	−0.58***
Central L	−0.34
Occipital L	−0.37
Alpha barycentric frequency	
Frontal R	0.53**
Central R	0.44*
Occipital R	0.27
Frontal L	0.58***
Central L	0.44*
Occipital L	0.28
Beta relative activity	
Frontal R	0.66***
Central R	0.23
Occipital R	0.11
Frontal L	0.65***
Central L	0.45*
Occipital L	0.36

R = Right; L = left. * $p < 0.05$; ** $p < 0.02$; *** $p < 0.01$.

Study 2

Patients with enlarged ventricles showed a preponderance of negative symptoms, a higher degree of social disability (table III) and a chronic course (suggested by a significantly longer duration of illness: 8.6 ± 4.9 vs 4.8 ± 4.0 years, $p < 0.02$) when compared to patients with normal ventricles.

As far as C-EEG data are concerned, beta relative activity was significantly lower in patients with enlarged ventricles on right frontal, left frontal and right central leads; alpha relative activity was significantly higher in these patients on the left frontal lead (table IV).

Table III. Clinical variables in patients with enlarged and normal ventricles

Variables	Enlarged ventricles (n = 13)	Normal ventricles (n = 37)
Scores on selected CPRS items (mean ± SD)		
Depersonalization	0.34 ± 0.61	0.48 ± 0.76
Feeling controlled	0.57 ± 1.19	1.12 ± 1.30
Disrupted thoughts	0.50 ± 0.78	0.59 ± 0.96
Ideas of persecution	0.96 ± 1.55	1.17 ± 1.64
Commenting voices	0.17 ± 0.36	0.39 ± 0.42
Other auditory hallucinations	0.61 ± 0.79	0.88 ± 1.24
Lack of appropriate emotion	1.07 ± 0.65	0.97 ± 1.29
Withdrawal	0.98 ± 1.52	0.47 ± 0.65
Scores on SANS subscales (mean ± SD)		
Alogia	3.27 ± 1.33*	2.37 ± 1.41
Avolition	2.63 ± 1.63	2.44 ± 1.29
Anhedonia	3.42 ± 1.44	3.26 ± 1.25
Affective flattening	3.28 ± 1.40**	2.19 ± 1.26
Attentional impairment	2.86 ± 1.16**	1.90 ± 1.25
Summary score	15.50 ± 5.03**	12.06 ± 3.53
Scores on selected DAS subscales (mean ± SD)		
Self-care	2.83 ± 2.38*	1.49 ± 1.32
Social withdrawal	3.83 ± 2.33	2.81 ± 1.65
Participation in household activities	4.12 ± 1.92*	2.75 ± 1.80
Heterosexual role	4.47 ± 2.35	3.16 ± 2.10
Social contacts	3.85 ± 2.16	2.96 ± 2.17
Work performance	4.35 ± 2.25*	2.79 ± 2.01
Interests and information	4.19 ± 2.34	3.05 ± 2.29
Behavior in crises and emergencies	4.15 ± 2.28**	2.20 ± 2.35
Summary score (section 1)	11.56 ± 5.43*	8.44 ± 3.91
Summary score (section 2)	29.03 ± 11.62***	19.27 ± 10.40

* $p < 0.05$; ** $p < 0.02$; *** $p < 0.01$.

Discussion

The enhancement of CSF NA concentration in schizophrenic patients had been previously reported by our group [15], as well as by other authors [38, 39].

The finding of an increased low voltage fast activity in schizophrenic patients, replicated by our group in different schizophrenic samples [24, 25, 32], is consistent with the results reported by other investigators [6, 23,

Table IV. Relative activity on C-EEG in the different leads in patients with enlarged and normal ventricles

C-EEG parameter	Enlarged ventricles (n = 6)	Normal ventricles (n = 15)
Delta relative activity		
Frontal right	30.9 ± 12.9	32.0 ± 9.3
Central right	27.5 ± 12.0	27.9 ± 10.4
Occipital right	15.7 ± 13.5	19.4 ± 9.6
Frontal left	31.5 ± 11.8	32.0 ± 12.1
Central left	26.6 ± 9.1	29.6 ± 9.6
Occipital left	14.7 ± 9.8	18.9 ± 11.0
Theta relative activity		
Frontal right	17.2 ± 4.8	20.7 ± 3.5
Central right	17.0 ± 3.9	19.1 ± 4.7
Occipital right	9.0 ± 3.8	12.9 ± 4.5
Frontal left	16.0 ± 2.4	19.8 ± 4.1
Central left	16.8 ± 2.5	18.7 ± 4.2
Occipital left	9.7 ± 3.2	11.2 ± 4.4
Alpha relative activity		
Frontal right	42.6 ± 14.1	30.9 ± 10.4
Central right	45.7 ± 11.7	38.0 ± 2.6
Occipital right	65.5 ± 17.6	52.1 ± 16.6
Frontal left	42.1 ± 13.8*	29.1 ± 10.2
Central left	44.8 ± 10.4	36.0 ± 11.7
Occipital left	64.1 ± 19.4	53.2 ± 19.0
Beta relative activity		
Frontal right	9.2 ± 0.9***	16.2 ± 6.0
Central right	9.8 ± 1.7**	14.9 ± 4.0
Occipital right	9.7 ± 3.6	15.5 ± 7.7
Frontal left	10.4 ± 2.8**	19.0 ± 11.9
Central left	11.7 ± 3.2	15.6 ± 4.6
Occipital left	11.4 ± 8.9	16.6 ± 11.7

* $p < 0.05$; ** $p < 0.02$; *** $p < 0.001$.

40]. Moreover, an increase in beta activity has also been detected in psychotic children and in children at high risk for schizophrenia when compared with normal controls [41, 42].

The interpretation of this finding is still very controversial. According to some investigators, beta activity increase is the result of continuous, intense, abnormal activation of the cortex by subcortical mechanisms [43]. Mednick [44] proposed the hypothesis that an inadequate hippocampus, exerting a less than normal inhibitory influence on the brain stem reticular formation, could contribute to the existence of a chronic state of hyper-arousal. A possible relationship between beta activity and arousal has been discussed by a number of authors [45, 46].

Nevertheless, the similarity between schizophrenics' beta activity and fast waves observed following the administration of barbiturates (narrow band fast activity) has suggested the possibility that both effects might be a correlate of impaired alertness [23].

Giannitrapani [47], utilizing the concept of 'scanning', notes that dur-ing 'diffuse' stimuli (e.g. white noise) there is an increase of beta activity which diminishes when the stimulus is 'structured'. Thus, 'increased beta activity may indicate a decrease in alertness and data processing rather than an increase' [48].

The conflict between the two interpretations might be only apparent. Tissot [49], comparing the effects of chlorpromazine and LSD on stimulus perception, finds that the former increases, while the latter reduces the stimulus perception threshold. He observes that chlorpromazine seems likely to lessen the stimuli meaning whereas with LSD all the stimuli may become significant, which, in terms of information processing, means that they become the equivalent of a white noise. Thus, 'this hyperafferentation is the functional equivalent of a deafferentation'.

The significant positive correlation between EEG beta activity and NA levels in the CSF found in our study would support the hyperafferen-tation hypothesis.

The further discussion of this point requires a brief description of Luria's model of 'the working brain' [17]. As is well known, Luria identifies three functional systems in the human brain: the first, involved in the regulation of consciousness and general arousal, includes the brainstem and the archipallium; the second, including the posterior areas of the two hemispheres (parietal, temporal and occipital cortex), is responsible for processing and storage of incoming information; the third, represented by the anterior part of the hemispheres, the frontal lobes, houses the neuronal programs for intentional behavior and for modulation of on-going behav-ior. The principal assumption of the model is that none of the single sys-tems is entirely responsible for any complex activity: each of them takes part in the organization of single activities and specifically contributes to the organization of an individual's behavior. Within this theoretical framework, the increasing evidence of a 'hypofrontal pattern' in schizophrenic patients is highly intriguing.

The hyperafferentation hypothesis, suggested by the EEG and biochemical data, could be explained by a decrease of the prefrontal inhibitory control mechanism: the processing of incoming information in lower structures, lacking integration and direction, loses its selectivity, yielding to the 'white noise' stimulation condition. A genetically determined precarious cooperation among the different functional blocks would be suggested by the presence of an increased beta activity in children at risk for schizophrenia. The psychotic decompensation might be the result of an excessive demand (such as an increased environmental stimulation) on any of the functional systems. On the other hand, the disclosure of a negative symptomatology following the neuroleptic treatment could be explained by the fact that the control of the positive symptoms (linked to a hyperactivity of the first and the second block) uncovers the preexisting negative ones, probably related to the hypofunction of the third system. The pronounced negative symptomatology observed in patients with enlarged ventricles might be explained by a limbic and diencephalic atrophy: such a condition would not determine the production of marked positive symptoms masking the negative ones.

The finding of a hyperstable slow alpha rhythm in treatment resistant schizophrenics [50], as well as our result of a higher alpha relative activity (of slow frequency) on the left frontal lead in patients with enlarged ventricles, might suggest an arrested development or a regression in this electrophysiological activity in some schizophrenics [23]. A parallel between electrophysiological activity and the myelination process of the prefrontal cortex could be proposed. The myelination process is not complete until after the teenage years and this observation has been discussed as a possible explanation for the tendency of schizophrenia to appear in late adolescence [19].

So far, EEG contributions to the generation of hypotheses concerning the pathogenetic mechanisms underlying schizophrenic disorders are not irrelevant. The quality of noninvasiveness of neurophysiological techniques is of great importance especially when repeated and extensive investigations are planned. Of course, the complexity and the heterogeneity of the disorders under investigation require a multidimensional approach in which the inclusion of a more specific assessment of frontal lobe functioning in groups of schizophrenics showing clinical and biological heterogeneity appears highly advisable.

References

1 Itil, T.M.; Saletu, B.; Davis, S.: EEG findings in chronic schizophrenics based on digital computer period analysis and analogue power spectra. Biol. Psychiat. *5:* 1–13 (1972).
2 Shagass, C.: An electrophysiological view of schizophrenia. Biol. Psychiat. *11:* 3–30 (1976).
3 Flor-Henry, P.; Koles, Z.J.; Sussmann, P.S.: Multivariate EEG analysis of the endogenous psychoses; in Perris, Kemali, Koukkou-Lehmann, Neurophysiological correlates of normal cognition and psychopathology. Adv. biol. Psychiat., vol. 13, pp. 196–210 (Karger, Basel 1983).
4 Shagass, C.: EEG and evoked potentials in the psychoses; in Freedman, Biology of the major psychoses. A comparative analysis, pp. 101–127 (Raven Press, New York 1975).
5 Mirsky, A.F.: Neuropsychological bases of schizophrenia. A. Rev. Psychol. *20:* 321–348 (1969).
6 Itil, T.M.: Qualitative and quantitative EEG findings in schizophrenia. Schizophrenia Bull. *3:* 61–79 (1977).
7 Crow, T.J.: Molecular pathology of schizophrenia: more than one disease process? Br. Med. *280:* 1–9 (1980).
8 Andreasen, N.C.; Olsen, S.A.; Dennert, J.W.; Smith, M.R.: Ventricular enlargement in schizophrenia: relationship to positive and negative symptoms. Am. J. Psychiat. *139:* 297–302 (1982).
9 Cross, A.J.; Crow, T.J.; Owen, F.: 3H-Flupenthixol binding in the brains of schizophrenics: evidence for a selective increase of dopamine D_2 receptors. Psychopharmacology *74:* 122–124 (1981).
10 Johnstone, E.C.; Crow, T.J.; Frith, C.D.; Husband, J.; Kreel, L.: Cerebral ventricular size and cognitive impairment in chronic schizophrenia. Lancet *ii:* 924–926 (1976).
11 Weinberger, D.R.; Bigelow, L.B.; Kleinman, J.E.; Klein, S.T.; Rosenblatt, J.E.; Wyatt, R.J.: Cerebral ventricular enlargement in chronic schizophrenia. An association with poor response to treatment. Archs gen. Psychiat. *37:* 11–13 (1980).
12 Ferrier, I.N.; Roberts, G.W.; Crow, T.J.; Johnstone, E.C.; Owens, D.G.C.; Lee, Y.C.; O'Shaughnessy, D.; Adrian, T.E.; Polak, J.M.; Bloom, S.R.: Reduced cholecystokinin-like and somatostatin-like immunoreactivity in limbic lobe is associated with negative symptoms in schizophrenia. Life Sci. *33:* 475–482 (1983).
13 Potkin, S.G.; Weinberger, D.R.; Linnoila, M.; Wyatt, R.J.: Low CSF 5-hydroxyindoleacetic acid in schizophrenic patients with enlarged ventricles. Am. J. Psychiat. *140:* 21–25 (1983).
14 van Kammen, D.P.; Mann, L.S.; Steinberg, D.E.; Scheinin, M.; Ninan, P.T.; Kammen, W.B. van; Linnoila, M.: Cortical atrophy and enlarged ventricles associated with low levels of cerebrospinal fluid monoamine metabolites and dopamine-beta-hydroxylase activity in schizophrenia; in Usdin, Carlsson, Dahlstrom, Engel, Catecholamines: neuropharmacology and central nervous system – therapeutic aspects, pp. 167–172 (Liss, New York 1984).
15 Kemali, D.; Del Vecchio, M.; Maj, M.: Increased noradrenaline levels in CSF and plasma of schizophrenic patients. Biol. Psychiat. *17:* 711–717 (1982).

16 Jackson, J.H.: Evolution and dissolution of the nervous system; in Taylor, Selected writings of John Hughlings Jackson, vol. II, pp. 45–53 (Hodder & Stoughton, London 1932).

17 Luria, A.R.: The working brain (Basic Books, New York 1973).

18 Ingvar, D.H.; Franzen, G.: Abnormalities of cerebral blood flow distribution in patients with chronic schizophrenia. Acta psychiat. scand. 50: 425–462 (1974).

19 Weinberger, D.R.; Faith Berman, K.; Zec, R.F.: Physiologic dysfunction of dorsolateral prefrontal cortex in schizophrenia. Archs gen. Psychiat. 43: 114–124 (1986).

20 Ingvar, D.H.: Functional landscapes of the dominant hemisphere. Brain Res. 107: 181–187 (1976).

21 Levin, S.: Frontal lobe dysfunctions in schizophrenia. II. Impairments of psychological and brain functions. J. psychiat. Res. 18: 57–72 (1984).

22 Abrams, R.; Taylor, M.A.: Differential EEG patterns in affective disorder and schizophrenia. Archs gen. Psychiat. 36: 1355–1358 (1979).

23 Giannitrapani, D.; Kayton, L.: Schizophrenia and EEG spectral analysis. Electroenceph. clin. Neurophysiol. 36: 377–386 (1974).

24 Kemali, D.; Vacca, L.; Marciano, F.; Nolfe, G.; Iorio, G.: C-EEG findings in schizophrenics, depressives, obsessives, heroin addicts and normals; in Perris, Kemali, Vacca, Electroneurophysiology and psychopathology. Adv. biol. Psychiat., vol. 6, pp. 17–28 (Karger, Basel 1981).

25 Kemali, D.; Maj, M.; Iorio, G.; Marciano, F.; Nolfe, G.; Galderisi, S.; Salvati, A.: Relationship between CSF noradrenaline levels, C-EEG indicators of activation and psychosis ratings in drug-free schizophrenic patients. Acta psychiat. scand. 71: 19–24 (1985).

26 Kemali, D.; Maj, M.; Galderisi, S.; Salvati, A.; Starace, F.; Valente, A.; Pirozzi, R.: Clinical, biological and neurophysiological features associated with lateral ventricular enlargement in DSM III schizophrenic disorder. Psychiat. Res. 21: 137–149 (1987).

27 Spitzer, R.L.; Endicott, J.; Robins, E.: Research diagnostic criteria (New York State Psychiatric Institute, New York 1975).

28 Asberg, M.; Montgomery, S.A.; Perris, C.; Schalling, D.; Sedvall, G.: A comprehensive psychopathological rating scale. Acta psychiat. scand., suppl. 271, pp. 5–27 (1978).

29 Da Prada, M.; Zurcher, G.: Simultaneous radioenzymatic determination of plasma and tissue adrenaline, noradrenaline and dopamine within the femtomole range. Life Sci. 19: 1161–1174 (1976).

30 Wurtman, R.J.; Axelrod, J.: A sensitive and specific assay for the examination of monoamine oxidase. Biochem. Pharmacol. 12: 1439–1441 (1963).

31 Winter, H.; Herschel, M.; Propping, P.; Friedl, W.; Vogel, F.: A twin study on three enzymes (DBH, COMT, MAO) of catecholamine metabolism. Correlations with MMPI. Psychopharmacology 57: 63–69 (1978).

32 Kemali, D.; Vacca, L.; Marciano, F.; Celani, T.; Nolfe, G.; Iorio, G.: Computerized EEG in schizophrenics. Neuropsychobiology 6: 260–267 (1980).

33 American Psychiatric Association: Diagnostic and statistical manual of mental disorders; 3rd ed. (Am. Psychiatric Ass., Washington 1980).

34 Kemali, D.; Maj, M.; Galderisi, S.; Ariano, M.G.; Cesarelli, M.; Milici, N.; Salvati, A.; Valente, A.; Volpe, M.: Clinical and neuropsychological correlates of cerebral ventricular enlargement in schizophrenia. J. psychiat. Res. 19: 587–596 (1985).

35   Andreasen, N.C.: Scale for the assessment of negative symptoms (SANS) (University of Iowa, Iowa City 1981).

36   Cannon-Spoor, H.E.; Potkin, S.G.; Wyatt, R.J.: Measurement of premorbid adjustment in chronic schizophrenia. Schizophrenia Bull. *8:* 470–484 (1982).

37   Jablensky, A.; Schwarz, R.; Tomov, T.: WHO collaborative study of impairments and disabilities associated with schizophrenic disorders. Acta psychiat. scand., suppl. 267, pp. 152–163 (1980).

38   Lake, C.R.; Sternberg, D.E.; Kammen, D.P. van; Ballenger, J.C.; Ziegler, M.G.; Post, R.M.; Kopin, I.J.; Bunney, W.E., Jr.: Schizophrenia: elevated cerebrospinal fluid norepinephrine. Science *207:* 331–333 (1980).

39   Gomes, U.C.R.; Shanley, B.C.; Potgieter, L.; Roux, J.T.: Noradrenergic overactivity in chronic schizophrenia: evidence based on cerebrospinal fluid noradrenaline and cyclic nucleotide concentrations. Br. J. Psychiat. *137:* 346–351 (1980).

40   Lester, B.K.; Edwards, R.J.: EEG fast activity in schizophrenic and control subjects. Int. J. Neuropsychiat. *2:* 143–156 (1966).

41   Simeon, J.; Saletu, B.: Neurophysiology and child psychiatry; in Saletu, Berner, Hollister, Neuropsychopharmacology, pp. 349–360 (Pergamon Press, Oxford 1979).

42   Itil, T.M.; Hsu, W.; Saletu, B.; Mednick, S.: Computer EEG and auditory evoked potential investigations in children at high risk for schizophrenia. Am. J. Psychiat. *131:* 892–900 (1974).

43   Hill, D.: Electroencephalography (MacDonald, London 1956).

44   Mednick, S.A.: Breakdown in individuals at high risk for schizophrenia: possible predispositional perinatal factors. Ment. Hyg. *54:* 50–63 (1970).

45   Dustman, R.E.; Boswell, R.S.; Porter, P.B.: Beta brain waves as an index of alertness. Science *137:* 533–534 (1962).

46   Hermelin, B.M.; Venables, P.H.: Reaction time and alpha blocking in normal and severely subnormal subjects. J. exp. Psychol. *67:* 365–372 (1964).

47   Giannitrapani, D.: Scanning mechanisms and the EEG. Electroenceph. clin. Neurophysiol. *30:* 139–145 (1971).

48   Lifshitz, K.; Gradijan, J.: Spectral evaluation of the electroencephalogram: power and variability in chronic schizophrenics and control subjects. Psychophysiology *11:* 479–490 (1974).

49   Tissot, R.: Epistemologia costruttivista delle sindromi schizofreniche; in Tissot, Introduzione alla psichiatria biologica, pp. 90–102 (Masson Italia, Milano 1979).

50   Flugel, F.; Itil, T.M.; Stoerger, R.: Klinische und electroencephalographische Untersuchungen bei therapieresistenten schizophrenen Psychosen; in Bradley, Flugel, Hoch, Neuropsychopharmacology, vol. 3, pp. 474–477 (Elsevier, Amsterdam 1964).

51   Greenblatt, M.: Age and electroencephalographic abnormality in neuropsychiatric patients: a study of 1,593 cases. Am. J. Psychiat. *101:* 82–90 (1944).

52   Ellingson, R.J.: The incidence of EEG abnormality among patients with mental disorders of apparently nonorganic origin: a critical review. Am. J. Psychiat. *111:* 263–275 (1954).

53   Jasper, H.H.; Fitzpatrick, C.P.; Solomon, P.: Analogies and opposites in schizophrenia and epilepsy. Electroencephalography and clinical studies. Am. J. Psychiat. *95:* 835–851 (1939).

54 Finley, K.H.: On the occurrence of rapid frequency potential changes in the human electroencephalogram. Am. J. Psychiat. *101:* 194–200 (1944).
55 Gibbs, F.A.; Gibbs, E.L.; Lennox, W.G.: The likeness of the cortical dysrhythmias of schizophrenia and psychomotor epilepsy. Am. J. Psychiat. *95:* 255–268 (1938).
56 Hill, D.: Electroencephalogram in schizophrenia; in Richter, Schizophrenia: somatic aspects, pp. 33–51 (Macmillan, New York 1957).
57 Kennard, M.A.; Schwartzman, A.F.: A longitudinal study of electroencephalographic frequency patterns in mental hospital patients and normal controls. Electroenceph. clin. Neurophysiol. *9:* 263–274 (1957).
58 Volavka, J.; Matousek, M.; Roubicek, J.: EEG frequency analysis in schizophrenia. Acta psychiat. scand. *42:* 237–245 (1966).

Prof. D. Kemali, MD, Clinica Psichiatrica, Primo Policlinico Universitario, Piazza Miraglia 2, I-80138 Napoli (Italy)

Giannitrapani, Murri (eds.), The EEG of Mental Activities,
pp. 182–200 (Karger, Basel 1988)

EEG Spectral Analysis in Psychopathology

Pierre Flor-Henry

Alberta Hospital Edmonton, Edmonton, Alberta, Canada

In the last few years important insights into the cerebral physiology of
healthy and psychiatrically ill populations have been derived from the
spectral analysis of the EEG, carried out during various mental states:
cognitive rest (eyes open or closed); verbal or spatial mentation; and in
different states, normal or pathologic.

Technical Aspects

Basar [1] gives a lucid exposition of the fundamental aspects of spectral analysis which he considers to be the most important technique in
time-series analysis. The EEG is a continuous voltage-time set, in effect a
multivariate time series.

Cross-correlation functions give a quantitative measure of the degree
of relatedness between 2 time series through time. Similarly the autocorrelation function is used for the statistical description of a single time series
and is derived by a time displacement of the original series and averaging
the product of the 2 values over the time interval. It is an average measure
(correlation) of the relationship between random processes at one instant
of time and those at another instant in time.

The power spectrum can be obtained by the Fourier transformation of
the autocorrelation function. The spectrum is the decomposition of a time
series into its sinusoidal components.

In essence, the Fourier transformation reduces complex functions to a
series of simple, sinusoidal waves. It transforms a continuous time series

into a discontinuous frequency spectrum which gives the average power distribution of a signal with respect to frequency. If the signal undergoes slow variations, it is concentrated at low frequencies. If it exhibits regular oscillations, it peaks at the fundamental frequency or at its harmonic frequencies; if it is randomly fluctuating, it is distributed over a broad spectrum.

The phase spectrum can be determined from the cross-correlation function if there is a correlation between 2 random processes. It appears in the form of a preferred phase angle related to frequency and estimates the degree to which an event systematically leads, or lags behind, another event.

The coherence function is derived from the power spectrum and the cross-spectrum of 2 random processes. If the 2 processes are identical the coherence is equal to unity at all frequencies. If they are totally independent processes, the coherence is zero. Coherence functions retain no phase information and consider only the relationship between 2 processes in terms of power at particular frequencies. Coherence, therefore, is a measure of the degree of statistical dependence of one set of events in relation to another set of events.

EEG Power and Coherence in Schizophrenia

Giannitrapani and Kayton [2] gave a full analysis of material first reported in 1971 in abstract form [3]. An interesting left lateralized finding emerged since in the log. amplitude analysis of *homologous* brain areas the controls were asymmetric with greater left temporal activation. This was not found in the schizophrenics. In their series of 10 young schizophrenics, some findings, partially confirmed by Itil et al. [4] and Lifshitz and Gradijan [5], were noted. They observed a significant increase in beta power, peaking at 19 and 29 Hz in all 16 monopolar derivations studied, together with a reduction in low beta power (10–18 Hz). The dominant alpha frequency (9 Hz) was significantly lower in the patients than in the controls (11 Hz).

Later, Giannitrapani [6] reported on the phase and coherence characteristics of the same subjects. The schizophrenics were found to have higher coherence than normals (particularly on the right) and a less pronounced T_3–T_4 left phase lead.

Lifshitz and Gradijan [5], in the spectral evaluations of the EEG of 30 male schizophrenics compared to an equal number of controls, found beta power significantly higher in the schizophrenics, particularly between 34- and 54-Hz frequencies, and the variability of the EEG was reduced in the 18- to 32-Hz range. The EEG derivations were unipolar left occipital and left paracentral.

In a first unpublished report in 1973 on 6 chronic schizophrenics, Etevenon found a reversal of right/left power peak values in the alpha frequencies following treatment with neuroleptics for 14 days. From the same laboratory Pidoux et al. [7] analyzed 57 EEG from 10 schizophrenics compared to 14 controls and, considering the alpha activity, found maximal hypovariability and highest power in the hebephrenics while the paranoids had the lowest amplitudes and greatest variability. Compared to the controls, the schizophrenics showed an increase in proportional alpha power in the left parieto-occipital derivation.

Etevenon et al. [8], still favoring the posterior cerebral regions, reported on the statistical characteristics of the EEG of schizophrenics compared to healthy controls. All EEG were administered in the relaxed, eyes-closed condition. The most powerful discriminator between the 2 groups was reduced alpha variability from the left centroparietal derivations, followed by a lowered (centroid) mean frequency (theta range) from the left parieto-occipital region in schizophrenia [9]. They [8] concluded that schizophrenics appear to fall into 2 distinct groups: one with high alpha amplitude (proportional alpha) including most hebephrenic forms and the other with low alpha amplitude close to the paranoid forms. In the high alpha group there is a relative reduction of peak alpha amplitude in the left hemisphere, and in the right hemisphere in the case of the low alpha category.

Stevens et al. [10] continuously recorded the EEG of 40 schizophrenics (most of whom were unmedicated) by radiotelemetry for periods ranging between 2 and 24 h. The schizophrenics had more delta and less alpha power than the controls. During hallucinations, the patients showed a reduction in left temporal power, accompanied by an increase in right temporal slow activity. Both the schizophrenics and the controls desynchronized in the left hemisphere during verbal tasks, but the schizophrenics, unlike the normals, also showed left hemisphere activation during spatial tasks. The 5 illustrative cases which Stevens and her colleagues detailed all had clear, lateralized EEG abnormalities localized to the left temporal lobe [11].

Stevens and Livermore [12] reported on telemetered EEG in a new sample of 18 essentially unmedicated schizophrenics who were compared to healthy controls. The patients showed 'a striking increase in left centro-parietal activity (slow)' during hallucinatory states. The pooled spectra from all the patients during all the abnormal (psychiatric) events compared to the pooled spectra of these patients when not victim of the psychopathological intrusions 'disclosed suppression of left temporal alpha during abnormal events'.

Coger et al. [13] compared the power spectral density patterns of 15 chronic schizophrenics (nonparanoid), unmedicated, with 15 age-matched normal controls, both groups consisting exclusively of males. There was a significant increase in power in the delta-theta range, bilaterally, and a left hemisphere energy increase in the 25- to 29-Hz frequencies, frontotemporally, in schizophrenia. This effect was principally due to the contribution from the schizophrenics with 'dominant hemisphere symptoms' (i.e. conceptual disorganization, grandiosity, anger, unusual thought content).

Abrams and Taylor [14] undertook a careful, blind visual evaluation of the EEG of 27 schizophrenics and 132 manic-depressive patients. In the manic-depressive group two thirds were manic and one third depressed. The incidence of EEG abnormality was lowest in depression (6.5%), intermediate in mania (16.8%), and highest in schizophrenia (25.9%). The EEG abnormalities were temporal in schizophrenia and parieto-occipital in the manic-depressive psychoses. There was a lateralization to the left hemisphere in schizophrenia and to the right hemisphere in manic-depressive syndrome. The EEG differences were unrelated to age, sex, and severity of illness or past or present drug administration.

In a study of EEG power and coherence Shaw et al. [15] compared the statistical EEG organization of 12 schizophrenics (on neuroleptic medication), 12 unmedicated neurotic depressives, and 12 healthy controls. The schizophrenics had significantly less alpha power in the left posterior-temporal derivation than the normals or neurotics. In the theta band, the neurotics differed significantly from normals and schizophrenics with a positive power ratio in contrast to the negative power ratio found in both normals and schizophrenics. Abnormal left hemisphere activation in schizophrenia and abnormal right hemisphere activation in the neurotic forms of depression are suggested by this investigation.

Fenton et al. [16] undertook the spectral analysis of 26 acute schizophrenics (inpatients), 30 chronic schizophrenics (outpatients), and 18 chronic hospitalized schizophrenics, whom they compared to each other and to a group of neurotic depressives (n = 31) as well as 2 normal control groups, young (n = 18) and old (n = 20). In the age-matched comparisons it was found that: (1) acute schizophrenics had less temporal alpha power than the controls; (2) there was a similar alpha power reduction in the chronic outpatient schizophrenics, extending to a power reduction in the low beta range; (3) the chronic hospitalized schizophrenics had a significant increase in power in the delta range (1–4 Hz) and in the low beta band (14–29 Hz).

EEG Studies in Unipolar and Bipolar Psychoses

For the last 15 years we have been engaged in the systematic analysis of the EEG, both in normal subjects and in various psychopathological syndromes, studied under various conditions: resting state, eyes open and closed, during verbal and spatial cognitive activation [17–19].

In 1980 we discussed the energy, coherence and phase characteristics of normals, depressives and manics [20]. In the normals cognitive activation (verbal and spatial) was associated with a reduction in absolute power in the alpha band and an increase in power in the beta bands. The logarithms of the right/left power ratios were task-dependent in the alpha band, an effect that became progressively weaker with increasing frequency and that was stronger in the parietal than in the temporal regions. The magnitude of the coherence measures during mental activity was reduced in all areas, except parietally where there was a significant increase in interhemispheric parietal coherence in the alpha band. The analysis of the right/left coherence ratios (intrahemispheric) revealed a task-dependent effect. On average, coherence over the cognitively activated hemisphere was greater than that of the nonengaged hemisphere. This was true for all frequencies.

We analyzed the statistical EEG patterns revealed by all the psychotics (all unmedicated) we had investigated to date: 63 psychotic depressions (unipolar and bipolar), 75 manias, and 53 schizophrenias [21]. These were compared to each other and in turn to 60 normal controls, all dextrals. The statistical comparisons (univariate) were undertaken for power, phase and coherence characteristics in the 8- to 13-Hz bands, composite power spectra having shown the complete absence of myogenic contamination of the EEG spectra for these frequencies. The results suggested the presence of increasing disorganization of the right hemisphere, least in depression, intermediate in mania and maximal in schizophrenia, together with left hemisphere disorganization in both mania and schizophrenia, again maximal in schizophrenia.

When we examined the EEG configurations in the bipolar psychoses (n = 78) compared to the unipolar psychoses (n = 55), the few statistical differences found were all related to the left parietal zone. The power and variance in this area were significantly reduced in the bipolar states (eyes closed) in the alpha frequencies. The logarithm of the right/left parietal coefficient of variation ratio was positive in unipolar and negative in bipolar psychoses. There were no significant differences between the 2 groups in the eyes open or in the verbal-cognitive conditions. During the spatial tasks the phase lead of the left parietal zone with respect to the right temporal region was significantly more pronounced in the bipolar syndromes.

A multivariate analysis restricted to the alpha frequency band was performed [22]. Coherence alone, interacting with the different cognitive states, provided the basis for the neurophysiological discrimination of the 3 psychoses from each other as well as from normal controls. The differentiation rested principally on coherence, highest in normals, intermediate in depressives, and smallest in manics and schizophrenics.

EEG Power Oscillations

Because of possible abnormalities of interhemispheric organization in the psychoses, we developed an EEG measure to estimate right/left hemispheric energy oscillations [23]. The average logarithm of the power ratios over 3-min epochs was calculated, from which at each sampling interval (15 times/s) the 'instantaneous' power ratio was subtracted, thus giving a measure of right/left hemispheric energy oscillations through time.

We examined the energy oscillations in the series of psychotics [21], considering only the alpha frequency band. We found that compared to controls (all dextral): schizophrenics had slower oscillations in the resting conditions and during both verbal tasks but normal oscillations during the spatial task. In depressives there were slower oscillations in both resting conditions and in both verbal tasks but normal oscillations in the spatial task. Manics had normal oscillations in both resting conditions, slow oscillations in both verbal tasks, and increased oscillations in the spatial task.

In the comparisons made between the psychotics: (1) schizophrenics had slower parietal oscillations than manics (eyes open, vocabulary); (2) depressives had slower parietal oscillations than schizophrenics (spatial); (3) manics had faster parietal oscillations than depressives (spatial). The exact interpretation of these complex relationships is at this stage uncertain. Nevertheless, the interaction between disturbed interhemisphere state and engagement of the left hemisphere (but not the right) in schizophrenia and depression is striking, as is the perturbation, in the opposite direction in mania, interacting with right (but not left hemisphere) processing.

Asymmetric Effects on EEG of Psychotropic Agents

We next studied the effect of lithium [24] in 12 normal healthy volunteers investigated in the same way, before and after one week of lithium carbonate treatment when the average plasma lithium level of the group was 0.86 mEq/l. There was no muscle artifact in any of the recordings analyzed, either before or after lithium. In the resting state lithium was associated with a significant increase in right parietal power in right parietal variance in the 20- to 50-Hz frequencies while the logarithm of the right/left parietal power ratio shifted from negative to positive.

In the frequency range in question, both these EEG events implied an activation of neural systems in the right hemisphere. Verbal cognitive activation, before and after lithium, was not associated with any statistically significant changes in EEG state. However, cognitive processing in the right hemisphere during spatial tasks (all subjects were 100% dextral) was profoundly affected by lithium. It produced an increase in right posterior temporal power (at T_6) in the alpha band and an increased intrahemispheric coherence in the left frontotemporal derivations (F_7–T_5), still in the alpha frequencies. The logarithm of the right/left posterior temporal power ratios went from negative to positive.

The parietal and frontal phase relationships were all reversed and opposite to those found before lithium during spatial processing (8–13 Hz) with phase lead in the right before and in the left after lithium. At rest, lithium slowed the temporal energy oscillations (8–13 Hz). These findings suggested that lithium, in normals, alters interhemispheric energy relationships in a complex manner that interacts with nondominant hemispheric systems and visuospatial processing.

By contrast Mori et al. [25] examined the effects of neuroleptics on the laterality of alpha activity at rest and during photic stimulation in 40 schizophrenic males and 20 normal volunteers, all dextral. Alpha amplitudes at rest and during photic stimulation were more prominent on the right side in normals and untreated schizophrenics. Medicated patients exhibited left-sided alpha dominance. In a second study [26] 19 alcoholics treated with phenothiazines and sulpiride showed, again, left-sided dominance, while with benzodiazepines right-sided dominance as in controls was found. Other studies reveal that psychotropic agents provoke bilaterally asymmetric effects on EEG organization. As early as 1973 Serafetinides [27] had shown that schizophrenics who recovered on phenothiazines exhibited left hemispheric EEG alterations.

In healthy normal subjects Laurian et al. [28] found there was also evidence of a left hemispheric bias in the distribution of dopamine since, following a single injection of chlorpromazine, predominantly left hemispheric changes occur in the power spectral EEG parameters. Von Knorring [29], administering imipramine to normal subjects, found a significant consequent increase in left frontal alpha power, i.e. corresponding to a state of right hemispheric activation.

EEG in Depression and Mania and during Positive and Negative Emotions

The quantitative EEG investigations of depression carried out by Prichep [30] showed that EEG parameters can correctly classify 84% of depressed subjects and 90% of the healthy controls. She studied 103 unmedicated depressed patients compared to 120 controls in the eyes closed condition.

In depression the following occurred: anterior coherence was reduced and absolute power in the fronto-temporal regions was increased as was power asymmetry. Total absolute power asymmetry, right > left was found in unipolar forms. Right temporal > left was found in bipolar psychoses which in addition exhibited left > right asymmetry in the central regions with unipolar leads. With bipolar montage and considering proportional power, unipolar depressions were characterized by slow-wave asymmetry (right > left). Bipolar depressions had the opposite asymmetry (left > right).

For the alpha frequencies, unipolars were either symmetrical or had increased power on the left, compared to the right, while the bipolars showed a suppression of left-sided alpha power. In the bipolar asymmetry of fast activity, right > left was also found. By discriminant function analysis an 85% correct classification of unipolar and bipolar was achieved. By utilizing the frontal coherence parameter alone there was a 70% correct differentiation of all depressives from the controls.

If one accepts the usual view that local neural activation is translated into local increases in EEG power in the slow and fast frequencies and a decrease in power in the alpha band, then right hemisphere activation is suggested, overall, in depression, particularly in the unipolar forms. Bipolar mood psychoses, compared to unipolar, have a greaer degree of left hemispheric changes. A general reduction of frontal interhemispheric EEG coherence is an important aspect of the EEG disorganization occurring in depressive psychoses.

The neurometric analysis of John et al. [31] leading (after z-transformation) to topographic maps confirms that the cross-spectral coherence matrix in the delta, theta, alpha and beta bands reveals significantly different patterns in unipolar and bipolar depressives, schizophrenics and normals.

Nystrom et al. [32] examined the relationships between EEG parameters and clinical characteristics in 25 patients with major depressive disorder before pharmacological treatment. Primary depression was associated with increased delta power and psychomotor retardation with increased delta and theta amplitudes. Recurrent unipolar depression was related to a decrease of total alpha power asymmetry. The left/right ratio of the mean integrated amplitude was negatively correlated with the severity of depression.

Davidson's [33] studies of regional EEG desynchronization during positive and negative emotions in full-term infants, 2 or 3 days old, and in 10-month-old infants indicated that relatively right fronto-parietal activation (3–6 Hz) during negative and left hemispheric activation (6–12 Hz) during positive emotions were already apparent.

In normal adults Davidson [33] reported that the alpha power lateralization ratios indicated relatively right frontal activation for negative and left frontal activation for positive emotions. Both positive and negative emotions, however, were associated with right parietal activation. In normal female dextral adults a pattern was found in which greater resting right frontal activation predicted those subjects who showed a greater intensity of fear responses when viewing disturbing films.

Comparing depressed with nondepressed adults Davidson [33] reported a pattern of diminished left frontal activation in the depressed group. The presence of reduced left frontal activation in depression was consistent with a disruption of dominant frontal inhibitory regulatory mechanisms provoking contralateral activation through disinhibitory release. In normals a tachistoscopic stimulus presented in the right visual field (i.e. to the left hemisphere) elicited greater positive affect than the same stimulus presented to the left visual field (right hemisphere). In depressed subjects the situation was reversed. In addition they produced more left frontal EEG activation to left visual field (right hemisphere) than to right field stimuli. Parietal EEG reactivity was the same in depression and controls and in the expected direction. The role of the right frontal system in the generation of dysphoric mood, fear, and negative emotions in normals clearly emerged in the systematic investigations of Davidson and his collaborators.

Cole and Ray [34] investigated 40 normal dextral males and found increased power in fast frequencies (16–24 Hz) more abundant during positive than negative emotional valence in the temporal and parietal regions, independent of hemisphere. Significant effects by hemisphere also emerged in the alpha and beta frequencies with, in all cases, greater power in the right hemisphere.

The EEG and auditory evoked potential study of Endo et al. [35] also implicated the right hemisphere in depression. The patients, cases of major depression with melancholia (unmedicated), and the controls were studied at rest with eyes closed. Peak alpha amplitudes were calculated frontally and parietally and parietal/frontal alpha amplitude indices were derived from the right and the left hemispheres. Depressed patients showed relative predominance of right frontal alpha amplitudes (relative to parietal) whereas the normals were symmetrical. For depressives the values were smaller than for the controls for both the right and left hemispheres, but for depressives this difference was significantly greater on the right than on the left. In the AEP study of these same depressed patients the P100-N100 amplitude (1,000-Hz tone) exhibited abnormal right intrahemispheric relationships compared with the controls with lower relative frontal amplitudes.

Considering our EEG findings in an earlier series on psychotic patients we [21] concluded: 'Given the importance of left brain inhibition of right brain neural systems mediating emotionality, sexual arousal and aggression a parsimonious hypothesis is to postulate a primary left temporal locus of dysfunction in psychosis. By disinhibiting the right hemisphere the symptomatology of depression is provoked. Mania results from an extension of this process which now disrupts right brain inhibition of left brain systems with consequent abnormal overactivation of the left hemisphere. At their most extreme intensity these perturbations of interhemisphere inhibitory systems are responsible for the symptomatology of acute schizophrenia.'

Recent Studies

In our most recent EEG studies of psychosis [36], we found that manics and depressives differed from normals in the resting conditions because of increased absolute power in the right fronto-temporal regions in the delta, theta and beta frequencies. Factored coherences in the delta, theta and alpha bands were significantly different in schizophrenics, manics, depressives and normals but only in the two resting conditions: eyes open and closed.

Examination of the canonical correlations indicated zones of power independence in the right hemisphere in depression and mania. A dislocation (absence) of normal antero-posterior power relationships was found in schizophrenic and manic psychoses. Complex changes in lateral and interhemispheric coherence relationships were seen in depressives, manics and schizophrenics when compared to each other and to normals. When clear, lateralized coherence configurations emerged distinguishing psychotics from normals, the right hemisphere was implicated in depression and mania and the left hemisphere in schizophrenia.

Ford et al. [37] studied power and coherence values in a variety of diagnostic groups: paranoid schizophrenics, dysthymic disorders, major affective disorders and a geriatric group. Some subjects were on neuroleptics or tricyclics; others were unmedicated. Coherence measures, usually in the alpha frequency band, were better discriminators between the groups than power measures. In these psychiatric groups paranoid schizophrenics had higher coherence. Coherence decreased with neuroleptics, decreased with age and increased with tricyclic antidepressants (the condition was eyes closed).

Takigawa [38] also noted a disruption of antero-posterior intrahemispheric coherence relationships in schizophrenics with incoherent speech.

Through generating 'EEG prints', analogous to voice prints which show changes in power as a function of time, he observed in these patients a disappearance of alpha power regularities and the emergence of abnormal irregular voltage in the beta frequencies.

Gaebel and Ulrich [39] examined alpha power characteristics in medicated schizophrenics at rest (eyes closed) and during visual motor tracking tasks. In both healthy controls and schizophrenics the performance of women was inferior to that of men. Patients with 'schizophrenia specific symptomatology' (i.e. with positive symptoms) were impaired on the visual tracking task whereas the 'withdrawal-retardation syndrome' had no impact on tracking performance [40]. Patients with more acute schizophrenic symptoms had greater relatively left hemispheric activation than those in remission in the resting state. Patients who did not improve on neuroleptics were in a state of relatively right hemispheric activation compared to treatment responsive patients [41]. Whereas in normals performance on the visual task related to right hemisphere activation, in the schizophrenics it was associated with relative activation of the left side. This last observation is in agreement with several previous results which showed a shift of cognitive lateral organization in psychosis [10, 20, 42].

The observation that treatment refractory patients had greater right hemispheric activation than those who became asymptomatic might suggest that, in the former, a more severe disturbance of dominant hemisphere function is associated with greater disruption of left brain inhibitory regulation of the right hemisphere. In addition, Gaebel and Ulrich [43] reported that schizophrenics with leftward gaze deviation had significantly more psychopathology than those with right gaze deviation.

Investigating EEG asymmetry in 10 schizophrenics, all males, before and after neuroleptic treatment, Merrin et al. [44] observed a significant reduction of right hemisphere alpha power in schizophrenia before treatment when compared to healthy controls. The log of the right/left power ratios of the patients after treatment did not differ from those of normals.

Scarone et al. [45], who examined unmedicated chronic and acute schizophrenics as well as the schizophrenia-spectrum type of personality disorders, restricted their EEG analysis to the parietal regions, right and left. They found a significant excess of fast activity in the left hemisphere of chronic schizophrenics and an excess of fast activity bilaterally in the acute group, which alone showed a reduction of alpha power in comparisons with the other diagnostic categories and the normal controls.

Ota et al. [46] analyzed 25 medicated schizophrenics with a special emphasis on positive and negative symptoms and their correlations with CT and EEG (alpha amplitude and peak). The sets of positive and negative symptoms were internally inter-correlated but the 2 sets were independent of each other in chronic schizophrenia: in acute schizophrenia, on the other hand, the sets were inter-correlated. Striking were the correlations between negative symptoms and cortical CT variables (i.e. Sylvian fissure dilatation and frontal lobe atrophy). Positive symptoms showed a negative correlation with occipital alpha amplitude while negative symptomatology was positively correlated with alpha amplitude.

Also implicating the left hemisphere in schizophrenia are the brain electrical activity mapping findings of Guenther et al. [47–49] who reported widespread hyporeactivity of the dominant hemisphere in type I schizophrenics when they performed simple and multisensory motor activity with their preferred (right) hand. With type II, deficit negative symptomatology schizophrenia, a bilateral hyporeactivity was found in delta, theta and beta frequencies – but not in alpha bands. In normals the amplitude of the contingent negative variation (CNV) was greater over the dominant than over the nondominant hemisphere and during verbal processes the left CNV was shifted more negatively than the right, even in the absence of overt speech.

Sato et al. [50], in the investigation of schizophrenics and controls, found in dextral subjects that both the resting CNV and that occurring after motor and verbal tasks were greater on the right side in schizophrenics. This reversal of CNV asymmetry was correlated with the following symptoms: apathy, blunted affect, thought disorganization and emotional withdrawal. The authors concluded that in schizophrenia there is impairment of those left thalamo-cortical projections that are related to verbal-linguistic processes.

Quantitative statistical EEG analysis also indicates the presence of abnormal neurophysiological configurations in sexual deviations. In the study of 39 exhibitionists compared to 19 normal controls matched for age, sex and handedness (20% sinistrality in the exhibitionists, all of whom were males) we found that a number of EEG parameters were significantly different in the two groups [51]. The essential characteristics of the exhibitionists were as follows: (1) reduced overall coherence; (2) slower oscillations; (3) reduced intra-hemispheric phase relationships, bilaterally;

(4) increased power (alpha); (5) smaller right/left frontal power ratio (alpha); (6) reduced left/right hemispheric phase lead. The significant differences were principally in the alpha frequency band.

Conclusion

It is clear that the statistical quantitative EEG analysis approach is, with increasing success in recent years, mapping the various patterns of cerebral disorganization which underlie psychopathological syndromes. EEG analysis will not be made obsolete by the exciting new technologies of brain imaging such as regional cerebral blood flow or positron emission tomography. It is more problematic at the level of spatial resolution but it is immensely superior in the area of temporal resolution.

By far the most frequently studied illness is schizophrenia. Given the heterogeneity of the syndrome, the variety of EEG parameters used, the different statistical analyses employed, pharmacological effects, the fact that the EEG signal is manifestly nonstationary (yet is treated as if stationary), that in the vast majority of studies to the distributions are not normalized (yet treated as if Gaussian), it is hardly surprising that many divergent and contradictory findings have been reported in EEG-schizophrenia research.

Certain convergent observations are of interest. The often made statement that schizophrenia is characterized by a significant reduction of alpha power is incorrect. It is only true for acute, positive symptomatology schizophrenia [8, 15, 43, 44]. On the other hand chronic schizophrenia with negative symptomatology is associated with an increase in alpha power [8, 44]. Numerous investigations document increased delta and beta activity in schizophrenia. Although complicated by the problem of eye-movement artifact (for delta) and myogenic infiltration of the EEG signal (for beta) and given the care with which many workers have attempted to remove artifacts, it is unreasonable to dismiss these repeated findings in schizophrenia as noncerebral in origin.

Asymmetric distribution in the beta frequencies, with a left-sided emphasis, has been observed in a number of studies of schizophrenic patients. A lateralized left-sided neurophysiological emphasis has been substantiated in 3 brain electrical activity mapping investigations [46, 52, 53].

There are reports of abnormal left hemisphere activation in schizophrenia, reflected by alpha power suppression on the left side (relative to the right). The work of Gaebel and Ulrich [39–41] indicates that acute, good prognosis schizophrenias are in a state of left- while chronic treatment-refractory forms are in a state of right-hemispheric activation. The right hemisphere alpha power suppression in schizophrenics before treatment, observed by Merrin et al. [44], can probably be understood in this perspective. It should be emphasized that the relationship between acute symptomatology, left-sided activation versus chronic, treatment refractory, right-sided activation schizophrenia described by Gaebel and Ulrich with respect to EEG parameters (and confirmed by visuo-motor effects and patterns of gaze deviation) coincides exactly with the dichotomy of florid symptomatology syndrome – electrodermal amplitude asymmetry (right < left) and chronic syndrome – electrodermal amplitude asymmetry (left < right) reported by Gruzelier [54]. I have discussed elsewhere [55] how these dichotomies are in turn related to bilaterally asymmetrical (left > right) hypermetabolic activity in acute and hypometabolic activity (left > right) in chronic forms of schizophrenia.

Mania has been neglected in quantitative EEG research, possibly because in most centers unmedicated manic patients are not available for study. In our investigations the patterns of EEG disorganization seen in mania are quite similar, in most respects, to those observed in schizophrenia but of lesser intensity and with more right-sided abnormalities.

Recently, depressive psychoses have been investigated by an increasing number of centers. EEG changes implicating the right hemisphere emerge quite strongly from this new body of evidence, particularly for unipolar depressive syndromes, together with a reduction of frontal coherence relationships. More left hemispheric abnormalities occur, however, in bipolar affective psychoses. In view of the progress made in the last 10 years in the field of quantitative EEG as applied to the study of psychopathology, it can be reasonably certain that in the very near future these neurophysiological techniques will be applied clinically and with therapeutic consequences in the objective definition of atypical psychoses.

References

1 Basar, E.: EEG – brain dynamics (Elsevier/North-Holland Biomedical Press, Amsterdam 1980).
2 Giannitrapani, D.; Kayton, L.: Schizophrenia and EEG spectral analysis. Electroenceph. clin. Neurophysiol. *36:* 377–386 (1974).

3   Giannitrapani, D.: Schizophrenia and EEG activity. Electroenceph. clin. Neurophysiol. *31:* 635 (1971).
4   Itil, T.M.; Saletu, B.; Davis, S.: EEG findings in chronic schizophrenics based on digital computer period analysis and analog power spectra. Biol. Psychiat. *5:* 1–13 (1972).
5   Lifshitz, K.; Gradijan, J.: Spectral evaluation of the EEG: power and variability in chronic schizophrenics and controls. Psychophysiology *11:* 479–490 (1974).
6   Giannitrapani, D.: Spatial organization of the EEG in normal and schizophrenic subjects. Electromyogr. clin. Neurophysiol. *19:* 125–145 (1979).
7   Pidoux, B.; Peron-Magnan, P.; Etevenon, P.R.; Verdeaux, G.; Deniker, P.: L'activité alpha dans un groupe de schizophrènes: analyse spectrale et comparison avec un groupe témoin. Rev. Electroencéphalogr. Neurophysiol. clin. *8:* 284–293 (1978).
8   Etevenon, P.R.; Peron-Magnan, P.; Campistron, D.; Verdeaux, G.: Changes in alpha amplitude in EEG's of schizophrenic patients compared to a control group; in Flor-Henry, Gruzelier, Laterality and psychopathology, pp. 269–290 (Elsevier, Amsterdam 1983).
9   Etevenon, P.R.; Peron-Magnan, P.; Rioux, P.; Pidoux, B.; Bisserbe, J.C.; Verdeaux, G.; Deniker, P.: Schizophrenia assessed by computerized EEG. Adv. biol. Psychiat. *6:* 29–34 (1981).
10 Stevens, J.R.; Bigelow, L.; Denney, D.; Lipkin, J.; Livermore, A.H., Jr.; Rauscher, F.; Wyatt, R.J.: Telemetered EEG-EOG during psychotic behaviors of schizophrenia. Archs gen. Psychiat. *36:* 251–262 (1979).
11 Flor-Henry, P.: Telemetered EEG in schizophrenia. J. Neurol. Neurosurg. Psychiat. *46:* 287 (1983).
12 Stevens, J.R.; Livermore, A.: Telemetered EEG in schizophrenia: spectral analysis during abnormal behaviour episodes. J. Neurol. Neurosurg. psychiat. *45:* 385–395 (1982).
13 Coger, R.W.; Dymond, M.; Serafetinides, E.A.: Electroencephalographic similarities between chronic alcoholics and chronic nonparanoid schizophrenics. Archs gen. Psychiat. *36:* 91–94 (1979).
14 Abrams, R.; Taylor, M.A.: Differential EEG patterns in affective disorder and schizophrenia. Archs gen. Psychiat. *36:* 1355–1358 (1979).
15 Shaw, J.C.; Brooks, S.; Colter, N.; O'Connor, K.P.: A comparison of schizophrenic and neurotic patients using EEG power and coherence spectra; in Gruzelier, Flor-Henry, Hemisphere asymmetries of function in psychopathology, pp. 257–284 (Elsevier/North-Holland Biomedical Press, Amsterdam 1979).
16 Fenton, G.W.; Fenwick, P.B.C.; Dollimore, J.; Dunn, T.L.; Hirsch, S.R.: EEG spectral analysis in schizophrenia. Br. J. Psychiat. *136:* 445–455 (1980).
17 Flor-Henry, P.; Koles, Z.J.; Bo-Lassen, P.; Yeudall, L.T.: Studies of the functional psychoses: power spectral EEG analysis. IRCS Med. Sci. *3:* 87 (1975).
18 Koles, Z.J.; Flor-Henry, P.: Mental activity and the EEG: task and workload related effects. Med. biol. Eng. Comp. *19:* 185–194 (1981).
19 Flor-Henry, P.; Koles, Z.J.; Howarth, B.G.; Burton, L.: Neurophysiological studies of schizophrenia, mania and depression; in Gruzelier, Flor-Henry, Hemisphere asymmetries of function in psychopathology, pp. 189–222 (Elsevier/North-Holland Biomedical Press, Amsterdam 1979).

20 Flor-Henry, P.; Koles, Z.J.: EEG studies in depression, mania and normals: evidence for partial shifts of laterality in the affective psychoses. Adv. biol. Psychiat., vol. 4, pp. 21–43 (Karger, Basel 1980).

21 Flor-Henry, P.; Koles, Z.J.: Statistical quantitative EEG studies of depression, mania, schizophrenia and normals. Biol. Psychol. *19:* 257–279 (1984).

22 Flor-Henry, P.; Koles, Z.J.; Sussman, P.: Multivariate EEG analysis of the endogenous psychoses. Adv. biol. Psychiat., vol. 13, pp. 196–210 (Karger, Basel 1983).

23 Flor-Henry, P.; Koles, Z.J.: Studies in right/left hemispheric energy oscillations in schizophrenia, mania, depressives and normals. Adv. biol. Psychiat., vol. 6, pp. 60–67 (Karger, Basel 1981).

24 Flor-Henry, P.; Koles, Z.J.: The effect of lithium on the EEG in mania and in normals. 3rd World Congr. of Biological Psychiatry, Stockholm 1981, abstract.

25 Mori, T.; Kato, H.; Kaiya, H.; Namba, M.: Neuroleptic effects on interhemispheric EEG amplitude. Folia psychiat. neurol. jap. *38:* 175 (1984).

26 Mori, T.; Kato, H.; Kaiya, H.; Nanba, M.: Neuroleptic effects on interhemispheric EEG amplitude (second report). Folia psychiat. neurol. jap. *39:* 104 (1985).

27 Serafetinides, E.A.: Voltage laterality in the EEG of psychiatric patients. Dis. nerv. Syst. *34:* 190–191 (1973).

28 Laurian, S.; Le, P.K.; Baumann, P.; Perey, M.; Gaillard, J.-M.: Relationship between plasma levels of chlorpromazine and effects on EEG and evoked potentials in healthy volunteers. Pharmacopsychiatria *14:* 199–204 (1981).

29 Von Knorring, L.: Interhemispheric EEG differences in affective disorders; in Flor-Henry, Gruzelier, Laterality and psychopathology, pp. 315–326 (Elsevier, Amsterdam 1983).

30 Prichep, L.: Neurometric quantitative EEG features of depressive disorders; in Takahashi, Flor-Henry, Gruzelier, Niwa, Cerebral dynamics, laterality and psychopathology, pp. 55–69 (Elsevier, Amsterdam 1987).

31 John, E.R.; Prichep, L.S.; Katz, J.; Easton, P.; Chabot, R.: Topographic maps of EEGs coherence and EP factor structure at rest and during mental tasks; in Takahashi, Flor-Henry, Gruzelier, Niwa, Cerebral dynamics, laterality and psychopathology, pp. 133–134 (Elsevier, Amsterdam 1987).

32 Nystrom, C.; Matousek, M.; Hallstrom, T.: Relationships between EEG and clinical characteristics in major depressive disorder. Acta psychiat. scand. *73:* 390–394 (1986).

33 Davidson, R.J.: Cerebral asymmetry and the nature of emotion: implications for the study of individual differences and psychopathology; in Takahashi, Flor-Henry, Gruzelier, Niwa, Cerebral dynamics, laterality and psychopathology, pp. 71–83 (Elsevier, Amsterdam 1987).

34 Cole, H.W.; Ray, W.J.: EEG correlates of emotional tasks related to attentional demands. Int. J. Psychophysiol. *3:* 33–41 (1985).

35 Endo, S.; Mori, T.; Mojima, D.; Akiyama, M.; Takagi, H.; Nuraoka, Y.; Kimura, M.: Quantitative EEG and evoked potential study on hemispheric differences in Japanese depressive patients; in Takahashi, Flor-Henry, Gruzelier, Niwa, Cerebral dynamics, laterality and psychopathology, pp. 85–92 (Elsevier, Amsterdam 1987).

36 Flor-Henry, P.; Koles, Z.J.; Lind, J.: Statistical EEG investigations of the endogenous psychoses: power and coherence; in Takahashi, Flor-Henry, Gruzelier, Niwa,

Cerebral dynamics, laterality and psychopathology, pp. 93–104 (Elsevier, Amsterdam 1987).

37 Ford, M.R.; Goethe, J.W.; Dekker, D.K.: EEG coherence and power in the discrimination of psychiatric disorders and medication effects. Biol. Psychiat. *21:* 1175–1188 (1986).

38 Takigawa, M.: A study of mutual correlation between EEGs of chronic schizophrenia with incoherent speech. Folia psychiat. neurol. jap. *38:* 175 (1984).

39 Gaebel, W.; Ulrich, G.: Visuomotor performance and alpha-power topography in the EEG: syndrome relationships in schizophrenia; in Takahashi, Flor-Henry, Gruzelier, Niwa, Cerebral dynamics, Laterality and psychopathology, pp. 161–172 (Elsevier, Amsterdam 1987).

40 Gaebel, W.; Ulrich, G.: Visuomotor performance of schizophrenic patients and normal controls. II. Results of a visual search task. Pharmacopsychiatry *19:* 190–191 (1986).

41 Gaebel, W.; Ulrich, G.: Topographical distribution of absolute alpha-power in schizophrenic outpatients – on drug responders vs. nonresponders. Pharmacopsychiat. *19:* 222–223 (1986).

42 Gur, R.E.; Skolnick, B.E.; Gur, R.C.; Caroff, S.; Rieger, W.; Obrist, W.D.; Younkin, D.; Reivich, M.: Brain function in psychiatric disorders. I. Regional cerebral blood flow in medicated schizophrenics. Archs gen. Psychiat. *40:* 1250–1254 (1983).

43 Gaebel, W.; Ulrich, G.: Visuomotor performance of schizophrenic patients and normal controls. I. Results of a visual fixation task. Pharmacopsychiatry *19:* 188–189 (1986).

44 Merrin, E.L.; Fein, G.; Floyd, T.C.; Yingling, C.D.: EEG asymmetry in schizophrenic patients before and during neuroleptic treatment. Biol. Psychiat. *21:* 455–464 (1986).

45 Scarone, S.; Gambini, O.; Colombo, C.; Cattaneo, R.; Bellodi, L.; Pugnetti, L.: Electrophysiological characteristics of hemispheric functioning in schizophrenic disorders: diagnostic and psychopathological correlates; in Takahashi, Flor-Henry, Gruzelier, Niwa, Cerebral dynamics, laterality and psychopathology, pp. 115–124 (Elsevier, Amsterdam 1987).

46 Ota, T.; Toyoshima, R.; Motomura, H.; Maeshiro, H.; Takazawa, A.; Ohshima, H.; Ishido, H.; Aikawa, H.; Tsukaha, Y.; Okada, S.; Yamauchi, T.: Biological heterogeneity of schizophrenia: morphological and psychophysiological evidence; in Takahashi, Flor-Henry, Gruzelier, Niwa, Cerebral dynamics, laterality and psychopathology, pp. 423–432 (Elsevier, Amsterdam 1987).

47 Guenther, W.; Breitling, D.: Predominant sensorimotor area left hemisphere dysfunction in schizophrenia measured by brain electrical activity mapping. Biol. Psychiat. *20:* 515–532 (1985).

48 Guenther, W.; Breitling, D.; Banquet, J.-P.; Marcie, P.; Rondot, P.: EEG mapping of left hemisphere dysfunction during motor performance in schizophrenia. Biol. Psychiat. *21:* 249–262 (1986).

49 Guenther, W.; Breitling, D.; Moser, E.; Davous, P.; Petsch, R.: Brain mapping rCBF and MRI measurements of motor dysfunction in type I and II schizophrenic patients; in Takahashi, Flor-Henry, Gruzelier, Niwa, Cerebral dynamics, laterality and psychopathology, pp. 519–533 (Elsevier, Amsterdam 1987).

50 Sato, Y.; Nakamura, M.; Takahashi, S.: Interhemispheric dysfunction on verbal task
    in schizophrenia; in Takahashi, Flor-Henry, Gruzelier, Niwa, Cerebral dynamics,
    laterality and psychopathology, pp. 239–244 (Elsevier, Amsterdam 1987).
51 Flor-Henry, P.; Koles, Z.J.; Reddon, J.R.; Baker, L.: Neurophysiological studies
    (EEG) of exhibitionism; in Shagass, Josiassen, Roemer, Brain electrical potentials
    and psychopathology, pp. 279–306 (Elsevier, Amsterdam 1986).
52 Morstyn, R.; Duffy, F.H.; McCarley, R.W.: Altered topography of EEG spectral
    content in schizophrenia. Electroenceph. clin. Neurophysiol. 56: 263–271 (1983).
53 Morihisa, J.M.; Duffy, F.H.; Wyatt, R.J.: Topographic analysis of computer pro-
    cessed electroencephalography in schizophrenia; in Usdin, Handin, Biological mark-
    ers in psychiatry and neurology, pp. 495–504 (Pergamon Press, Oxford 1982).
54 Gruzelier, J.H.: Hemispheric imbalance masquerading as paranoid and unparanoid
    syndromes? Schizophrenia Bull. 7: 662–673 (1981).
55 Flor-Henry, P.: Cerebral dynamics, laterality and psychopathology: a commentary;
    in Takahashi, Flor-Henry, Gruzelier, Niwa, Cerebral dynamics, laterality and psy-
    chopathology, pp. 3–21 (Elsevier, Amsterdam 1987).

P. Flor-Henry, MD, Alberta Hospital Edmonton, PO Box 307,
Edmonton, Alberta T5J 2J7 (Canada)

Subject Index